EFFECT OF HATHA Y´

PHYSIOLOGICAL

SHIV KANT

TABLE OF CONTENTS

Acknowledgement		*i*
List of Tables		*iii-vi*
List of Figures		*vii-viii*
CHAPTERS	**TOPIC**	**PAGE NO.**
I	**INTRODUCTION**	**1-24**
	• Statement of the problem	19
	• Objectives of the study	20
	• Hypotheses of the study	20
	• Delimitations of the study	21
	• Limitations of the study	22
	• Definitions/explanations of the terms used	22
	• Significance of the study	24
II	**REVIEW OF RELATED LITERATURE**	**25-56**
III	**METHOD AND PROCEDURE**	**57-92**
	• Design of the study	57
	• Selection of subjects	58
	• Selection of variables	58
	• Selection of tests	60
	• Orientation of the subjects	61
	• Instrumental reliability	62
	• Reliability of the data	62
	• Pilot study	63
	• Training programs	63
	• Administration of tests	84
	• Collection of data	91
	• Statistical Procedure	92
IV	**ANALYSIS OF THE DATA, RESULTS AND DISCUSSION**	**93-156**
	• Data analysis and results of the study	93
	• Discussion on findings	150
	• Testing of hypotheses	153
V	**SUMMARY, FINDINGS, CONCLUSIONS AND RECOMMENDATIONS**	**157-163**
	• Summary	157
	• Findings	157
	• Conclusions	161
	• Recommendations	162
BIBLIOGRAPHY		**164-174**
APPENDICES		**175-194**

LIST OF FIGURE

SR. NO.	TITLE	PAGE NO.
3.1	Flow chart showing the methodology adopted in this study.	57
3.2	The detailed distribution of the sample	58
3.3	Flow chart showing the experimental treatment adopted for experimental group –I.	64
3.4	Tad asana performed by Asana group	66
3.5	Trikonasana performed by Asana group	66
3.6	Padmasana performed by Asana group	66
3.7	Vajrasana performed by Asana group	67
3.8	Bhujangasana performed by Asana group	67
3.9	Salabhasana performed by Asana group	67
3.10	Dhanurasana performed by Asana group	68
3.11	Halasana performed by Asana group	68
3.12	Chakrasana performed by Asana group	68
3.13	Matsayasana performed by Asana group	69
3.14	Flow chart showing the experimental treatment adopted for experimental group –II.	69
3.15	Bhastrika performed by Pranayama group	70
3.16	Kapalbhati performed by Pranayama group	71
3.17	Anulom Vilom performed by Pranayama group	71
3.18	Shitali performed by Pranayama group	71
3.19	Bhramari performed by Pranayama group	72
3.20	Udgeeth performed by Pranayama group	72
3.21	Flow chart showing the experimental treatment adopted for experimental group –III	73
3.22	Tad asana performed by asana and pranayama combined group	74
3.23	Padmasana performed by asana and pranayama combined group	74
3.24	Bhujangasana performed by asana and pranayama combined group	75
3.25	Salabhasana performed by asana and pranayama combined group	75
3.26	Halasana performed by asana and pranayama combined group	75
3.27	Bhastrika performed by asana and pranayama combined group	76
3.28	AnulomVilom performed by asana and pranayama combined group	76
3.29	Udgeeth performed by asana and pranayama combined group	76
3.30	50 meter dash run test	84
3.31	Broad jump test	85

SR. NO.	TITLE	PAGE NO.
3.32	Shuttle run test	86
3.33	Sit and reach test	86
3.34	12 Minutes run/walk test	87
3.35	Systolic and diastolic blood pressure measurement	88
3.36	Resting heart rate measurement	89
3.37	Breath holding time measurement	90
3.38	Blood test	91
4.1	Mean speed for 50 Meter Dash Run in pre-test and post-test among various groups	96
4.2	Estimated marginal means of 50 meter dash run	99
4.3	Pre and post test comparison for strength during standing broad jump	101
4.4	Estimated marginal means of broad jump	103
4.5	Pre and post test comparison for agility through Shuttle run (seconds)	105
4.6	Estimated marginal means of shuttle run	107
4.7	Pre and post test comparison for flexibility through Sit and reach(cm)	109
4.8	Estimated marginal means of sit and reach	112
4.9	Pre and post test comparison for Endurance through 12 minute walk/run(meter)	114
4.10	Estimated marginal means of 12 minutes run/ walk during post-test	116
4.11	Pre and post test comparison for Systolic Blood pressure	119
4.12	Adjusted mean plot for systolic blood pressure	121
4.13	Pre and post test comparison for diastolic Blood Pressure	123
4.14	Adjusted Mean Plot for Diastolic Blood Pressure during post-test	125
4.15	Pre and post test comparison for Heart rate	127
4.16	Adjusted Mean Plot for resting heart rate during post-test	129
4.17	Pre and post test comparison for breath holding capacity	131
4.18	Adjusted Mean Plot for Breath Holding Capacity	134
4.19	Pre and post test comparison for White Blood cells	136
4.20	Adjusted Mean Plot for White Blood Cells	138
4.21	Pre and post test comparison for Red Blood cells	140
4.22	Adjusted Mean Plot for Red Blood Cells of Different Groups	142
4.23	Pre and post test comparison for Hemoglobin	144
4.24	Adjusted Mean Plot for Hemoglobin of Different Groups	146
4.25	Pre and post test comparison for Hemoglobin	148
4.26	Adjusted Mean Plot for Platelets	150

LIST OF TABLES

SR. NO.	TITLE	PAGE NO.
3.1	Selected Variables, Units, Tests & Equipments	61
3.2	Reliability co-efficient of physical fitness parameters	62
3.3	Reliability co-efficient of physiological parameters	63
3.4	yoga asana training detailed program	65
3.5	Pranayama group training program	70
3.6	Asana and pranayama combined group training program.	73
4.1	Mean speed for 50 m dash (Second) run among groups in pre-test.	94
4.2	Pre and post-test comparison for speed through 50 mts dash (seconds)	95
4.3	Descriptive Statistics of Groups without Adjustment of Mean speed	96
4.4	Levene's Test of Equality of Error Variances	97
4.5	Analysis of Covariance for Post Intervention speed (50 Meter Dash run)	97
4.6	Post Hoc Analysis for Speed 50 Meter Dash run (Seconds)	98
4.7	Average strength during broad jump (meter) by groups in pre-test	99
4.8	Pre and post-test comparison for strength during Broad jump (mts)	100
4.9	Descriptive Statistics for without Adjusted Mean strength	101
4.10	Equality of Variance among Groups for Standing Broad Jump	102
4.11	Analysis of Covariance for Post Intervention Standing Broad Jump	102
4.12	Post-hoc Analysis for Strength(Standing Broad Jump)	103
4.13	Average agility while Shuttle Run(seconds) among groups in pre-test	104
4.14	Pre and post-test comparison for agility through Shuttle run (seconds)	104
4.15	Statistics for without Adjusted Mean agility during post-test	106

SR. NO.	TITLE	PAGE NO.
4.16	Equality of Variance among Groups for Shuttle Run in post-test	106
4.17	Analysis of Covariance for Post Intervention Agility(Shuttle Run)	106
4.18	Post Hoc Analysis for agility Shuttle run (seconds)	107
4.19	Average flexibility for sit and reach(cm.) among groups in pre-test	108
4.20	Pre and post-test comparison of Flexibility Sit and reach (cm)	108
4.21	Descriptive Statistics of Flexibility (Sit and Reach(cm.)) without Adjusted Mean	110
4.22	Equality of Variances among Groups regarding Flexibility(Sit and Reach(cm.))	110
4.23	Analysis of Covariance among Groups for Post Intervention Flexibility (Sit and Reach(cm.))	111
4.24	Post Hoc Analysis for Flexibility(Sit and Reach(cm)) during post-test	111
4.25	Average pre-test endurance for 12 minute walk/run(meter)	112
4.26	Pre and post-test comparison of endurance(12 minutes walk run (m))	113
4.27	Descriptive Statistics of Endurance(12 minutes walk run (m)) without Adjusted Mean	114
4.28	Equality of Variance for Endurance(12 minutes walk run (m))	115
4.29	Analysis of Covariance among Groups for Post Intervention Endurance (12 minutes walk run (m))	115
4.30	Post Hoc Analysis for Endurance (12 minutes walk run (m)) during post-test	116
4.31	Average SBP among groups in pre-test	117
4.32	Pre and post-test comparison of SBP (mm/Hg)	118
4.33	Descriptive Statistics of Groups without Adjustment for Mean Systolic Blood Pressure	119
4.34	Equality of Error Variance among Groups for Systolic Blood Pressure	120
4.35	Analysis of Covariance among Groups for Post Intervention Systolic Blood Pressure	120

SR. NO.	TITLE	PAGE NO.
4.36	Average Diastolic Blood pressure(mmHg) among groups in pre-test	121
4.37	Pre and post comparison of Diastolic Blood pressure (mm Hg)	122
4.38	Descriptive Statistics of Diastolic Blood pressure(mm Hg) without Adjusted Mean	123
4.39	Equality of Error Variance among Groups in their Diastolic Blood Pressure	124
4.40	Analysis of Covariance among Groups for Post Intervention Diastolic Blood Pressure	124
4.41	Average Heart rate among groups in pre-test	125
4.42	Pre and post comparison of HR (per minute)	126
4.43	Descriptive Statistics of Groups without Adjusted Mean for Resting Heart Rate	127
4.44	Equality of Error Variance among Groups in their Resting Heart Rate	128
4.45	Analysis of Covariance among Groups for Post Intervention Resting Heart Rate	128
4.46	Post Hoc Analysis of Heart rate (per minute)	129
4.47	Average breath holding capacity(seconds) among groups in pre-test	130
4.48	Pre and post comparison of breath holding capacity(seconds)	130
4.49	Descriptive Statistics of Breath Holding Capacity without Adjusted Mean	132
4.50	Equality of Error Variance of Breath Holding among Groups	132
4.51	Analysis of Covariance among Groups for Post Intervention Breath Holding Capacity	133
4.52	Post Hoc Analysis of Breath Holding Capacity(seconds)	133
4.53	Mean WBC(10^3/uL)among groups in pre-test	135
4.54	Pre and post comparison of WBC(10^3/uL)	135
4.55	Descriptive Statistics of White Blood Cells without Adjusted Mean	137
4.56	Equality of Error Variance of White Blood Cells among Groups	137

SR. NO.	TITLE	PAGE NO.
4.57	Analysis of Covariance of White Blood Cells after Adjusted Mean among Groups	137
4.58	Mean RBC(10^6/uL)among groups in pre-test	139
4.59	Pre and post comparison of RBC (10^6/uL)	139
4.60	Descriptive Statistics of Red Blood Cells without Adjusted Mean	141
4.61	Equality of Error Variance of Red Blood Cells among Groups	141
4.62	Analysis of Covariance or Red Blood Cells after Adjusted the Mean	142
4.63	Mean Hemoglobin(g/dL) among groups in pre-test	143
4.64	Pre and post comparison of Hemoglobin (gm/dL)	143
4.65	Descriptive Statistics of Hemoglobin of Respondents of Different Groups	145
4.66	Equality of Error Variance of Hemoglobin among Groups	145
4.67	Analysis of Covariance for Posttest of Hemoglobin with Covariate of Pretest among Different Groups	145
4.68	Mean Platelets(10^3/uL) among groups in pre-test	146
4.69	Pre and post comparison of Platelets(10^3/uL)	147
4.70	Descriptive Statistics of Platelets of Respondents at their Post Phase of Measurement without Adjusted Mean	148
4.71	Equality of Error Variance of Platelets	149
4.72	Analysis of Covariance for Platelets after Adjusting Mean	149

CHAPTER-I

INTRODUCTION

"Action is movement with intelligence; the world is filled with movement.

What the world needs is more conscious movement, more action".

- (B.K.S. Lyengar)

During the last few decades, the life style of the people has totally changed. The way of life and other social systems have changed greatly throughout the world. There is a lot of competition for survival in this modern world. Everyone is on peak in materialistic sense. Our present educational system has failed to achieve the ultimate aim of education. Today, the main aim of the students is collecting degrees and diplomas only.

Most of the youngsters and children have become patients due to different conditions of life and work culture. They are not spared from the stress and strains of life. They live in a hurry-up world of busy parents, incessant lessons, video games and irregular eating habits. They are not aware about their mental and physical fitness. It is very difficult to stay healthy due to a large number of problems in routine life.

We all are looking towards yoga for solving to various health problems which are common in this modern world. Thus yoga is a combination of discipline and art which directly affects the existence of man at every level. Therefore, the importance and need of yoga must be felt in every sphere of life. It develops the whole personality of an individual like physical, mental, moral and intellectual.

So, this study was conducted to know the effects of hatha yoga on physical fitness, physiological and haematological variables of school level students.

Yoga is a very archaic regulation. It is appreciable as a great influential tradition of India. Yoga is a way to wisdom with healthiness and satisfaction. Yoga assists to make one"s life (the result of intentionally planning and trying something), useful and noble. The remuneration of yoga helps every part of each stage. „Silencing of the mind`s activities which lead to complete realization of the native nature of the Supreme Being" **(Ross, 1993).**

Yoga is a historical foundation for healthiness and happiness in life. It is very helpful for harmony of mind and the body. Yoga is the way of becoming physically and mentally wellbeing. It contemporizes the function of the muscle and the mind. It is a path that can lead us towards health **(Batch, 1987).**

Yoga is not a very old story buried in nothingness. It is the most valuable and important need of today and the culture of tomorrow **(Satyananda, 1969).**

It is a mode of existence (life). It is a perfect procedure to educate our body, mind and inner spirit. This is an art of best living which was practised in India thousands of years ago but as yoga deals with full harmony of life; its instructions are applicable today as they were in the primordial period. Some people think yoga belongs to one religion but its benefits were experienced by the Buddhists, Jews, Muslims, Christians, Hindus and the Atheists also. Yoga is in unification together with each and every one **(Kindersley, 1996).**

„Our ancestors developed yoga towards combination of the body, intellect and spirit, the same time as harmonious complete" **(Satyananda, 1969).**

Yoga is a science and method of precise living. It is working on each and every aspect of human beings life: the bodily, very important intellectual and emotional **(Satyananda, 1969).**

"Where there is yoga, there is prosperity, success, freedom and bliss".

-B.K.S. Lyengar

YOGA:

Yoga is the best method in present days for healthy life. The word yoga comes from the Sanskrit word "yuj" which means join, unite, harness, and "yoke"**(Satyananda, 1969).**

In ancient India yoga implied joining or integrating all aspects of life of an individual like physical, mental and spiritual. The roots of yoga originated in ancient India. In oral traditions of yogis the knowledge of yoga was first passed by Lord Shiva to the lives of men.

Yoga is also referred in pre-Vedic Indian tradition and also mentioned in Rig-Veda. Yoga is also referred broadly in Hindu Upanishads but the origin of yoga to be much older than that. The chronology of earliest text describing yoga- practices is unclear, varyingly credited to the Upanishads **(Singleton, 2010).**

There are six famous branches of yoga:

Bhakti yoga: This branch of yoga mostly used in India as a path of heart and devotion.

Raj yoga: This branch of yoga is related to self-control. Yogis considered it as the king of yoga. Raj yoga practitioners achieve self-respect by learning to be masters.

Jnana yoga: this branch is related to mind. Yogis who practice this branch focus on mind, intelligence, wisdom and knowledge.

Karma yoga: karma yoga is related to service. Yogis related to this branch believed that one"s present situation was based on his past action. If we are doing selfless service in present, our future will be free from negativity and selfishness.

Tantra yoga: This branch of yoga is mostly misunderstood of all the paths. Tantra yoga is related to using rituals in order to experience what is scared.

Hatha yoga: It is the most popular branch of yoga. This branch of yoga includes physical poses or asanas and pranayama.

HISTORY OF YOGA:

According to the period of time the history of yoga is presented in different forms related to different situations of that time.

Pre- Vedic Period:

„Yoga may have pre- Vedic elements" **(Crangle, 1994).** Some positions of yoga originated in the Indus Valley Civilization. The Pashupati seal discovered in an Indus Valley Civilization location depicts a shape in a position similar to an asana used for meditation, Mulabandhasana.

Vedic Period (1700-500 BCE):

The source of knowledge: Vedas are a collection of hymns and rites which contain a comprehensive key to cosmic evolution. The oldest known yogic teachings and other related information"s are present in Vedas which is called Vedic yoga. Vedic yoga was used for reuniting the visible material world with the spiritual world. During Vedic period, gurus taught the people how to live in divine harmony, understanding the world. The term „yoga" was first used in the Rig-Veda which dates back to approximately 1500 before the Common Era; Rig-Veda is a collection of hymns and different ways of meditation. „The earliest evidence of yogis and yoga tradition is found in the Kes`in hymn 10.136 of Rigveda" **(Karel, 1977).**

Pre-Classical Period (500-200 BCE):

The pre-classical yoga period was the period of the creation of the Upanishads and early Buddhist texts **(Lerson, 2008).**

In this period systematic yoga concepts began to emerge in the texts. Approximately 200 scriptures describe the idea of karma and the cycle of birth and death. It"s also explains the relationship between (Brahma) and (Atman). Bhagavad-Gita was also created in this period. In the Bhagavad-Gita three aspects of life which are very important for our existence are:

1. **Bhgati (Gayan)**
2. **Knowledge**
3. **Cause and effect (Karma).**

These all three aspects search the sacrifice of the ego through self-knowledge.

In this time yoga was very important for Buddhism too. "The Buddha was the founder of his (Yoga) system, even though, admittedly, he made use of some of the experiences he had previously gained under various Yoga teachers of his time" **(Werner, 1998).**

The main cause of people`s suffering is desire, greed and delusion. Yoga lays stress on the importance of meditation and asana for a happy life. It is a method to achieve harmony of life. Yoga prevents our body and mind from bad situations and unhealthy lifestyle.

Classical Period – (200BCE-500 CE)

"(Yogas` citta- vrtti- nirodhah)".

- (Yoga sutras, 1.2)

Patanjali composed „Yoga sutra" in the classical yoga period. In Patanjali Yoga Sutra Yoga is presented in a very systematic and approachable way. Because of this wonderful work Patanjali has often been called the founder of Yoga. Patanjali believed that we are composed of Prakrti (Nature) and spirit from the material world. There are 195 sutras in yoga sutra which explain yoga in very detail.

In yoga sutra Patanjali expounded the practice of yoga into eight path of self-superiority.

1. **Yam** – Self-restraint- It is related to behavioral commitments. These commitments are Ahinsa (nonviolence), Satya (honesty), Asteya (non- stealing), Brahmacharya (celibacy) and Apaertigraha (non-hoarding).
2. **Niyama** - Observance of ethical code – Sauch (purity, cleanliness), Santosh (contentment), Tapas (persistent meditation), Svadhyaya (study of self), Ishvara Pranidhana (true self) **(Tummers, 2009).**
3. **Asana** - Physical posture – A position used for meditation. (Patanjali`s sutras)
4. **Pranayama** - Breath control
5. **Pratyahara** - Abbreviation of senses
6. **Dharana** - Concentration or focus
7. **Dhayana**–Meditation (control over sense organs)
8. **Samadhi** - Blissful awareness

If these eight stages of yoga are followed and practiced by man there would be an all-round development in life – physically, intellectually and spiritually and man would attain physical and mental equanimity **(Iyengar, 1963).**

Most of the yogis focused on meditation and ignored the other concepts of yoga in classical yoga period.

Post-Classical Yoga-

In the past yogis had paid much attention on meditation and spiritual part of yoga. They were not much interested in physical body. In post classical period yoga masters started to give main attention to the physical body with deep breathing and meditation.

Hatha yoga emerged in this period **(Larson, 2008).** Yoga masters began to probe the hidden powers of human body. This system would help to improve the physical body, prolong life and enlightenment. In this post classical yoga period there was a big change in yoga because of a dramatic increase in yogic literature.

Modern Yoga-

In this period of yoga a large number of yoga gurus including swami Vivekananda contributed a lot - other important yoga gurus include Swami Paramahansa yogananda, Swami Sivananda Radha, Swami Satchidananda and Maharishi Mahesh Yogi. Dalai Lama is a great yogi from Tibet in this period. He was a noble prize winner for peace and inspired many people to learn a about Buddhism and yoga. In modern age yoga Swami Sivananda presents the fire important principles of yoga-

1. Proper Relaxation
2. Proper Exercise
3. Proper Breathing
4. Proper Diet
5. Positive thinking & Meditation

In this age a number of yoga schools or styles are present in society. Swami Ram Dev is a very popular yoga guru at present time. Yoga is not a form of religion now. It is a philosophy of life. It is based on scientific facts. The main aim of yoga is development of total personality. It creates a proper balance between the body and the mind. Hatha yoga is the most famous form of yoga to achieve good body posture and peace of mind.

Hatha yoga

The origins of hatha yoga have come to the light in the eleventh century A.D. The word "hatha" derived from Sanskrit two words- ha and tha, "ha" means sun and "tha" means moon. It"s also called sun-moon yoga. It helps to strike a balance between opposite parts of the individual`s body like front and back, left and right. Hatha Yoga uses physical resources in order to achieve proper self development. Some yoga experts or yogis claimed that hatha yoga was developed by experts to help the people to remain healthy during the spiritual dark periods. „In India hatha yoga is firstly related to Natha Sampradaya" **(White & Gordon, 2012).**

Hatha yoga consists of eight limbs of practices but mainly concentrated on two limbs of the eight paths. These two paths were posture and breathing. Yoga teacher believes pranayama to be the most important for our body metabolic function. In a day we breathe roughly 23000 per day and use about 4500 gallons of air, which increase during exercise.

Thus breathing exercise is very important to health. Our prana or life force is directly related to our breath. We do not achieve optimal health and full potential of life if we breathe incorrectly. Pranayama is the science of correct breathing. It teaches us how to control the life force. In pranayama we practice breathing correctly and deeply.

On the other hand yoga asana (posture) are very helpful to improve flexibility, balance and strength in our body. Each asana has a definite form and steps for improving the desired position of the body. Yoga asana and pranayama scientifically developed the health and increase the strength of all parts of the body. These both types of exercise improve muscular tissue to glands and internal body organs.

Hatha yoga helps us to make strong and physically fit as any other exercise program. We enjoy all the benefits of asana with safe and regular practice of them. They bring spiritual power in the body and mind. Asana are very helpful to control inner energy. Regular practice of yoga prevents us from various diseases including cancer, diabetes, high or low blood pressure, kidney failure and mental disorder. It has developed into a – based physical fitness, stress- relief and relaxation technique **(Burley, 2000).**

Yoga is a way to achieve perfect balance and harmonizing the body emotion. Yogasana, breathing exercises, bandha practices, shatkarma are the parts of yoga. We realize the higher perception of life with systematic practice of them. Yoga facilitate to make one`s life focused, useful and noble. Thus yoga is a discipline which influences the progress of our day to day harmony to the human beings by physical practices with or without a toner on spiritualism. Hatha yoga emphasizes our physical health more than other yoga civilization **(Paul, 1982).**

There are two main limbs of Hatha yoga:

- **Asana**
- **Pranayama**

Asana:

An asana is a body posture. It is also defined as a sitting meditation pose. But in hath yoga and modern yoga it"s present as pose or position may be standing, inverted and twisting. Patanjali mentions the asana as one of the eight limbs of his system. According to yoga sutras asana is a position that is steady and comfortable. Asana also known as yoga poses or yoga postures in English. In Hatha Ratnavali provides a list of 84 asanas.

Yoga Asana are classified in to three main groups-

1. Asana used for meditative purpose- These postures are used for meditation. These types of asana are sitting on the floor. Padmasan (Lotus posture), siddhasana, Gomukhasana and Vajrasana etc are example of meditative asanas. The features of these asanas are:

1. Broad base
2. The buttocks or knees in horizontal plane
3. Head, neck and trunk are in a line and balancing condition
4. This is a steady and comfortable posture

2 Asana for relaxation and release of muscular tension:

Savasana and makrasana can be recognised as this type of asana. These postures release body tension and awareness of the whole body with lightness and a kind openness from with outward.

3. Corrective asana:

These asana are used for correcting musculoskeletal system. A large number of postures fall in this group. The salient features of this type asanas are following.

1. Asanas concerned to joints of body e.g.-Garudasana
2. Asana related to the vertebral Columns e.g. Salabhasana, Dhanurasana, Vakrasana

3. Asanas concerned with balancing of body: Mayurasana

This type of asanas produces Physiological balance in all the body system in the human body. It also helps to train the spinal cord and digestive system can work elastic. These asanas provide efficient exercise to abdominal muscle. Asanas like bhujangasana, Paschimotanasana and halasana are the examples of this type of postures.

Asanas were claimed to give both spiritual and physical benefits in medieval hatha yoga texts. More recently, studies have provided facts that they develop flexibility, strength, and balance; to decrease stress and conditions related to it; and specifically to alleviate some diseases **(Ross & Thomas, 2010).**

Pranayama:

"Tasmin Sati Shvasa Prashvsayoh Gati Vichchhedahb Pranayamah".

(Patanjali`s Yogasutra, 2.49)

Pranayama is a Sanskrit word which means "extension of the Breath or life force" the word pranayama composed of two words Pran which means life force and ayama means to control. Prana is the first expression of life. "Expansion of individual energy into cosmic energy is called pranayama" **(Mishra).**

Breath is produced by the motion of lungs. The ancient yogis used many types of breathing exercises to maximize the result of pranayama. We cannot survive more than a few minutes without our air. If we stop breath, life ends. The great yogis developed a unique system, Pranayama. It helps to increase, develop and control this life force. It helps to control our breath in a superior and extra ordinary way to achieve maximum benefits. Pranayama is a breathing training. It is the perfect method to synchronize all the organs of our body. It is the right way to mastering vitalizing effect on the body mind and spirit. Pranayama has three aspects the first is inhalation, the second is exhalation and the third is fixedness or suspension of breath **(Bhattacharyya, 1999).**

The main three components of pranayama are:

- **Poraka** – To inhale the breath
- **Kumbhaka-** Retain the breath
- **Rechaka** – Exhale the breath

Pranayama is directly related to "control of breath", Control the life force by awareness and coordinated breathing. With regular practice of pranayama we decrease in the number of respiration made per minute.

"When breath is irregular, your mind is also unsteady. But when your breath is still, so is your mind and you living long".

(Hatha Yoga Pradipika, 2.2)

Pranayama teaches us to breathe in a right way. We all can breathe but right method of breathing increases our lung capacity. It improves the quantity of air inhaled and exhaled and also helps to teach one"s body to work in harmony. Pranayama is very useful and helpful part of their training. Because breathing rhythm and more quantity of air means more stamina. When we are able to intake more air then we can get more oxygen every breath.

Our one third of lungs remains unutilized because of our shallow breathing. With the help of Pranayama we learn the deep breathing techniques and utilize our lungs to breathe effectively. It helps to intake more oxygen supply to our body, all the various organs and system work much more efficiently. It also helps to burn more body fat and digestion power also improves. Our immune system also strengthens because the flow of oxygen is increased. Pranayama helps to increase the expansion and contraction of our lungs so that they become capable for purifying more and more blood.

In other types of sports and exercise breathing is fast but not deep. Different types of wastes and impurities accumulate in innermost parts of body because oxygen does not reach these parts properly. After some time it seems as disease. With the help of Pranayama we purify and throw waste products out of the body.

BENEFITS OF YOGA:

Physical, Physiological and haematological Benefits of yoga:

In this modern and competitive world it is a big problem is hard to find time for physical activities. But all the people want to stay in perfect body structure. We all know about the importance of exercise in our daily life. Yoga is also simply, a seated training which is very beneficial for health and athletic ability. Regular yoga practice makes our body strong and flexible. Asana improves the stretching and relaxing ability of muscles and is very helpful for skeletal system of human body. This reduces the risk of injuring ligaments and tendon. **(Mallinson & Singleton, 2017)**

Yoga is also helpful for gently stretching of joints and ensures the optimum blood supply to every cell of body. Yoga improves the power of synchronization of the body and mind by systematically contracting and slaying muscle in the coordinate manners.

Continuing yoga exercise is the ideal complement to other type of systems of exercises like running; cycling and weight training. In yoga practice the body works systematically. The entire major muscle groups are used.

Yoga Asana improves the strength of different body parts like back, neck, shoulders, deep abdominal, and buttocks muscles. It is a fantastic strengthening practice. It`s help for building core strength of body. Yoga enhances your functionality in everyday life. It also brings nourishment to internal organs of body. „Yoga asana are the physical postures and exercises which tone up and make strong the internal and outer organs of the body‟ **(Mallinson & Singleton, 2017).**

All sports build your muscular strength and stamina in specific area. Yoga can also help to balance your muscular development and enable your body to function more efficiently. It‟s helps in relieving physical tension and improves our concentration and poise. Yoga also helps in enhancing your sports performance.

Yoga exercises helps to improve balance, focus and coordination of body There are plenty of yoga asanas which are beneficial for improving balance. Regular practice of yoga improves your concentration that will serve you in everyday life.

„Yoga is a system of self- renewal of total personality. It`s helpful in acquiring all round development of body. Through yoga we can achieve inner beauty and great spiritual peace‟ **(Kumar, 1992).**

Asana is the third limbs of Astang yoga. It is also called posture. A steady and good posture is very helpful to produces mental and physical equilibrium. It is not only a gymnastic exercise. With the help of postures we exercise every muscle, nerve and glands of body. We discipline our mind, reduce fatigue and relax the nerves with regular exercises of yoga Asana **(Lyengar, 1963).**

There is a number of physical benefits of yoga asana. We use all the muscles of body to hold and balance the poses. So it keeps our body strong. The yogic exercises and breathing practices improve our flexibility of joints and our muscles stay stronger. People suffering from a number of diseases like osteoarthritis or rheumatoid arteries" will see a noticeable improvement in their condition by continuous practice of yoga asana.

Yoga improves not only outer parts but also improves the functions of our inner systems of body like respiratory, circulatory, digestive and glands etc. It is also helpful in emotional control and stability of mind. With regular practice of yoga you can rebalance your body and take control on emotions.

It also creates a sense of calmness and well-being. Yoga activities are very beneficial for massages of all glands and inner organs. It stimulates the organs and keeps away the diseases. It is helpful in kicking out the toxins and providing nourishment to all parts of the body. These effects of the yoga leads to delayed ageing and improve the energy level of the body **(Newcombe, 2019).**

It allows us to balance the physical, mental and emotional stress. Yoga is the best therapeutically technique for many life style related problems. Balanced development of personality and emotional attitude of a person helps him to live happily and in co-ordination with environment. We can achieve biological equilibrium and tuning by doing yogic exercises.

Our heart works for all the 24 hours and does not take rest even for a single moment. Our lungs intake oxygen for purify the blood. In digestive system our stomach, liver and other glands play main role for the digestion of food. Regular exercises of yoga asanas are very beneficial for all above internal organs to function properly **(Sharma, 1984).**

Medical experts noted during research that in the absence of regular physical exercises, a chalk impurity is found in the muscles and other internal organs. It contains dangerous chemical substances like lime-phosphate and magnesia. This impurity is like poison for our body. It may be able to damage several part of human body. It affects the circulation of blood because it contracts the veins and arteries. But if we do yoga exercises daily, we can reduce the bad chemicals of our body and enhance our physical and mental fitness and increases the joy of healthy long life span **(Hayes & Chase, 2010).**

Systematic yoga exercises result in a good many changes in the body. These changes take place on the levels of cellular, tissues, organs and body structures. It also enhances cellular metabolic processes and the molecular mechanism and functional capacities of organs and their systems. Yoga asana helps to comfort of body function and also regulate the hormonal regulation and neural regulation. It also enhances muscular activity. Yoga is very useful for bio-chemical variable of our body. It"s very helpful for maintaining the quantity of glucose, sodium, cholesterol, triglycerides, catecholamines, total white blood cell and also increases the level of cholinesterase, A.T.P., hemoglobin, lymphocyte, vitamin, total protein etc. **(Broad, 2012).**

Regular yoga exercises have great impact on body composition and basic metabolic rate of our body. Our team body tissue is made of muscles, bones and other body organs. There are three types of fat tissues in our body.

- Essential fat
- Storage fat
- Non-Essential fat

Essential and storage fat are very helpful for body to function. Non-essential fat have no real time purpose. Yoga exercises have isometric resistance which helps us to build lean tissue in our body. It"s very helpful in building muscle. it maintains the whole body function smoothly.

Obesity is the main problem at this time. It"s the excessively high amount of body fat in relation to lean body mass. But cholesterol itself is not bad. It is group of a substances used by our body to keep us healthy. There are two types of cholesterol, good and bad. We need to understand the difference between them. Cholesterol is dangerous and creates problems when someone gets too much in one"s food. The extra amount of cholesterol can lead to block our arteries.

There are two important types of lipoprotein

1. High Density Lipoproteins (HDL)
2. Low Density Lipoproteins (LDL)

Low Density Lipoproteins are dangerous to our health because it causes blood vessels to clog and inhibits blood from flowing freely through the vessels. High Density Lipoproteins are known as „good"" because its helps to carry the cholesterol back to liver for re-processing.

In blood cholesterol combines with certain proteins and forms lipoproteins. Surya namaskara (A Dynamic series) is very helpful for the treatment and control of obesity. With the help of this dynamic series of asanas we produce all the good effects of exercises because it includes asana, pranayama, mantra and meditation. It is a complete practice in itself. It has a great effect and influence on the endocrine and our nervous system.

PHYSICAL FITNESS:

Some people use fitness as the synonym for health. But fitness is the ability of a person to function effectively and live zestfully. It is the sum of physical, mental, emotional, social and spiritual components. These all components of fitness are related to each other. It is also termed as "Total fitness". Physical fitness is the one aspect of total fitness. It would include ability of functioning of body organs. A physically fit individual has adequate level of muscular strength, endurance, co-ordination, flexibility and balance.

Physical fitness is the capacity of an individual to perform the routine work and special task effectively. When we reach a good physical fitness level, we realise that it"s most important for full growth and development **(Mathews, 1958)**.

A physically fit individual is more efficient to work hard and hard. He has the capacity to recover fast from fatigue. It"s a very common thing that if we want to enjoy a healthy life and physical fitness we engage ourselves to well coordinated rhythmical movements which is very helpful for organic and functional promotion of the body. Physical fitness is our ability to strive and live effectively with full adjustment with our environment and nature. Our satisfactory level of fitness depends upon regular participation in physical activities **(Tancred, 1987)**.

Many research reports strongly support that regular participation in yoga helps us to keep healthy and prevents from many diseases. It also helps to keep our heart strong. Regular exercises also enhance the capacity of oxygen consumption. We produce more energy because our metabolic process works in a healthy way. Physical fitness is our basic need. It is an important part of life. In every moments of life we need to be physically active. We can perform our best and effectively when we are physically fit. It helps to perform better in daily life style, sports and other activities.

VARIABLES OF THE STUDY:

To know the effects of Hatha yoga on school level students total 100 students were selected by researcher. They were divided in equal four groups. Each group had 25 students. In this study three type of hatha yoga trainings were used.

- **Asana Training (AT)**
- **Pranayama Training (PT)**
- **Asana And Pranayama combined Training (APT)**

First group was assigned for Asana training, second group for Pranayama training and the third group for asana and pranayama combined training. Fourth group was treated as control group. Duration of training was 12 weeks. Pre and post tests were conducted to know the effects of trainings.

Three types of dependent variables were selected. These all variables are very important for physical fitness and health.

- **Physical fitness variables.**
- **Physiological variables.**
- **Haematological variables.**

Physical fitness variables: -

Physical fitness refers to highest functional capability of all system of the body. We are exercising each time we move and keeping our body tuned and in a good running order. The body of human is framed in such a way that it can jump, climb, bend, stretch and do more tedious work. The human body becomes stronger as it exerts more and muscles participation matters a lot in shaping it. "Physical fitness is a set of attributes that are either health- or skill-related". **(Caspersen et al., 1985)**

Exercise helps in improving our health and builds up our energy and endurance. Yoga has very beneficial effects on our physical fitness variables. To know the effects of hatha yoga following physical fitness variables was selected:

Speed:

„Speed is the process of an athlete sprinting in order to cover distances in the shortest amount of time possible" **(Bompa & Buzzichelli, 2019).** Speed is the main component of fitness. It is the ability to move quickly. It is very important for success in many sports like sprint in track and field, cyclists and speed skaters etc. Speed is the key of success in many field team sports. It is also very important in overall fitness.

Strength:

It is the ability to carry out work against a resistance. Strength improves the quality of life and enhances the ability to do everyday activities. It`s also a main component of our performance in sports such weight lifting, wrestling and throwing. „Greater muscular strength is directly related with improved force-time characteristics that contribute to an athlete"s overall performance" **(Suchomel et al., 2016).**

Agility:

Agility is the ability to move and change direction fast. It helps in performance in sports activities like squash, tennis and many team games. It is the combination of speed, strength and body control.

Flexibility:

Flexibility is the range of motion for a given joint. It is directly influenced by muscles and connective tissues of the joint. Flexibility offers many physical benefits. It is an important component of fitness. It improves mobility and reduces the risk of injuries. A good flexibility of joints increases the neuromuscular coordination and blood supply to joint structures. Lack of flexibility may also lead to abnormal stress on our body joints and become cause of tendonitis. „Increasing the range of motion creates good posture and develops proficient performance in everyday activities increasing the length of life and overall health of the individual" **(Barratt, 1964).**

Endurance:

Endurance is the ability of muscles to repetitive motions without getting tired. It is the main component to improve performance in our sports and exercise activities. It is also very important for daily tasks. „A well trained athlete can be defined as, the athlete who executes his or her technique consistently and effectively with the least effort" **(Michael, 2008).**

Physiological Variables:

Physiology is the science of working of body and its organs. It is a branch of biology. Physiological effects of yoga are well known; physiological variables are one of the most important factors that determine the health level of an individual. The following physiological variables were selected for the present study.

Blood Pressure (Systolic and Diastolic blood pressure):

Systolic blood pressure is the force which heart exerts on arteries when it beats and Diastolic blood pressure is the force of heart exerts in between beats. Blood pressure range directly affects our health. Normal range of blood pressure is 120/80 mm/hg **(Caro, 1978).** Now a day"s high blood pressure and low blood pressure is very common. Both situations are very dangerous for our health.

Resting Heart Rate:

It is the number of times your heart beats per minutes when you are completely at rest. It also shows your heart fitness level. A lower resting heart rate is better when it is due to your good health. It shows that your heart pumps more blood with each contraction. It gives more rest to your heart and is a sign of healthy heart.

Breath Holding Capacity:

It is a test to measure respiratory endurance. It improves our breathing and lungs functions. It also shows the fitness level of your lungs and working level of your respiratory system.

Haematological variables

Haematological methods are widely utilised as a means for individual health assessment. The following haematological variables were selected to know the effect of hatha yoga.

White blood cells:

It`s also called leukocytes. These are the cells of immune system. They protect our body against infectious diseases. These cells are formed in bone marrow. WBC`S are very essential for health because they are most important part of our immune system. Leukocytes are found throughout the body, including the blood and lymphatic system. White blood cells compose approximately 1% of the total blood volume in a healthy adult **(Maton et al., 1997)**.

Red blood cells:

Red blood cells carry fresh oxygen throughout the body. It is a main component of our blood. These cells are very important to our health. Red blood cells have hemoglobin which carries oxygen. Red blood cells are extremely flexible and deformable so as to squeeze through minute capillaries, as well as to maximize their apposing surface by assuming a cigar shape, where they competently release their oxygen load. Red blood cells also help to remove carbon dioxide from body **(Goodman et al., 2007)**.

Haemoglobin:

Haemoglobin is protein found in red blood cells that carries oxygen in your body and it gives red colour to blood. It is essential for our body to transferring oxygen in tissues. It is also directly related to our health. So it is very important content in our blood. „Hemoglobin also carries the essential regulatory particle nitric oxide bound to a globin protein thiol group, releasing it at the same time as oxygen" **(Epstein & Hsia, 1998)**.

Platelets:

Platelets are very small blood cells. It`s shaped like a disc. It plays important role in making our blood thicker. If our blood vessels are damaged platelets form clots to stop bleeding. They are made in our bone marrow **(Machlus et al., 2014)**. Its normal count is 150,000 to 450,000 per micro liter of blood.

IMPORTANCE OF THE PRESENT STUDY:

Man`s life has become very fast, busy and full of tension due to great development of science and technology. Our physical work has been largely taken away by the machines. But due to technology the pressure on the nerves has greatly increased. Physical, physiological and psychological processes of body are disturbed. The reason behind it is lack of regular physical activity and mental tension. This situation makes very negative impact on the organs and glands. Our real basis on this earth is physical; if we are physically weak then we will not be able to face the problems in life.

School level students are the foundation of our society. They also face this challenge of inactivity. Most of their time is spent on computers, study and video games. We need one such instrument for them which can develop them fully and enhance their personality.

Yoga is the best way to keep them active and healthy. It is one of the best methods used for physical and mental health development. So there is a great need of yoga and yogic exercises to be taught to the students. It helps them to overcome physical, physiological and haematological problems.

A lot of researches were conducted on effects of yoga at higher level of age and different types of diseases. But very few studies were conducted at school level students. This study is a scientific support to benefits of yoga on physical fitness, physiological and haematological variables of school level students.

This study supports that children should do yoga exercises daily so that they can remain physically healthy. Schools should give proper place to yoga in schools along with other sports. This study also helps in designing the training programs of yoga for school children that can have maximum beneficial effects on their health.

STATEMENT OF THE PROBLEM:

The title of the problem has been stated as ***"EFFECT OF HATHA YOGA ON PHYSICAL FITNESS, PHYSIOLOGICAL AND HAEMATOLOGICAL VARIABLES OF SCHOOL LEVEL STUDENTS."***

OBJECTIVES OF THE STUDY:

1. To ascertain the effects of asana training, pranayama training and asana & pranayama combined training on physical fitness variables of their respective group.
2. To find out that which training has better effects on physical fitness variables within asana training, pranayama training and asana & pranayama combined training.
3. To ascertain the effects of yoga asana training, pranayama training and asana & pranayama combined training on physiological variables of their respective group.
4. To find out that which training has better effects on physiological variables within asana training, pranayama training and asana & pranayama combined training.
5. To ascertain the effects of yoga asana training, pranayama training and asana & pranayama combined training on haematological variables of their respective group.
6. To find out that which training has better effects on haematological variables within asana training, pranayama training and asana & pranayama combined training.

HYPOTHESES OF THE STUDY:

On the basis of literature reviewed and scholar`s own understanding of the problem, the following **Null Hypotheses** were formulated**:**

1. There would be no significant difference in physical fitness variables on yoga asana group, pranayama group and asana & pranayama combined group due to their respective hatha yoga trainings.
2. It was hypothesized that asana training, pranayama training and asana & pranayama combined training equally effects the physical fitness variables of their respective group.

3. There would be no significant difference in physiological variables on yoga asana group, pranayama group and asana & pranayama combined group due to their respective hatha yoga trainings.
4. It was hypothesized that asana training, pranayama training and asana & pranayama combined training equally effects the physiological variables of their respective group.
5. There would be no significant difference in haematological variables on yoga asana group, pranayama group and asana & pranayama combined group due to their respective hatha yoga trainings.
6. It was hypothesized that asana training, pranayama training and asana & pranayama combined training equally effects the haematological variables of their respective group.

DELIMITATIONS OF THE STUDY:

1. The study was delimited to 100 students of Govt. Sr. Sec. School Ugalan District Hisar, Haryana, India only.
2. The study was delimited to 9th to 12th class Students only.
3. The study was delimited to male students only.
4. The study was delimited to Yoga asana, pranayama and their combinations of exercises.
5. The experimental period was delimited to 12 weeks.
6. The training was delimited to five day in a week.
7. The study was delimited to the following physical fitness variables:
   - Speed
   - Strength
   - Agility
   - Flexibility
   - Endurance

8. The study was delimited to the following physiological variables:
   - Systolic blood pressure
   - Diastolic blood pressure
   - Resting heart rate
   - Breath holding capacity
9. The study was delimited to the following haematological variables: -
   - White blood cell
   - Red blood cell
   - Hemoglobin
   - Platelets count.

LIMITATIONS OF THE STUDY:

The following points were considered as limitations of the present study

1. Atmosphere, climatic conditions and percentage of humidity were uncontrollable factors during the training period.
2. Food habits, life style and health conditions of the subjects during yoga training and testing period were not controlled.
3. Activities other than the training schedule of the subjects were not fully controllable.
4. Family problems.
5. During the training period, the aptitude of the students might influence the results. So aptitude of the subjects was considered as one of the limitation of the study.

DEFINITIONS/EXPLANATIONS OF THE TERMS USED:

- **Yoga-** According to Panini, the term yoga can be derived from either of two roots, *yujir yoga* (To yoke) or to yuj samadhau ("to concentrate") **(Dasgupta, 1975).**
- **Asana-** The Yoga Sutras of Patanjali define "asana" as "[a position that] is steady and comfortable". Patanjali mentions the ability to sit for extended periods as one of the eight limbs of his system.

- **Pranayama-** Pranayama comes from 2 Sanskrit words –Prana (life force) and Ayama (control). So, in its complete description, Pranayama would mean the control the flow of breath. To most, control of breath is Pranayama **(Macdonell, 1996).**

- **Physical fitness-** Physical fitness is one"s ability to execute daily activities with optimal performance, endurance, and strength with the management of disease, fatigue, and stress and reduced sedentary behavior **(Campbell et al., 2013).**

- **Strength** – Strength is the force that a muscle or a muscle group can produce against resistance in one maximal effort **(Gothi, 1993).**

- **Speed** – Speed is the ability to move quickly across the ground or move limbs rapidly to grab or throw **(Wood, 2010).**

- **Flexibility** – „Flexibility is the ability of a joint or muscle to move through its full range of motion" **(Wood, 2010).**

- **Agility:** Rapid whole body moment with change of velocity or direction in response to a stimulus **(Sheppard and Young, 2006).**

- **Endurance** – "Endurance is the ability of an organism to exert itself and remain active for a long period of time, as well as its ability to resist, withstand, and recover from fatigue" **(Encyclopedia.com).**

- **Breathe holding capacity-** A rough index of cardiopulmonary reserve measured by the length of time that a person who is a study subject can voluntarily stop breathing **(Farlex Partner Medical Dictionary).**

- **Pulse rate** – Pulse rate is the rate of beats of the heart per minute. It is measured by tactile or visual means on the outside of an artery **(Zhang & Zhang, 2009).**

- **Blood pressure** – It is a force that moves blood into arteries and drains blood from the arteries as blood moves through the circulatory system **(Ignasiak, 2007).**

- **Red blood cells** – it is also called erythrocyte. It carries oxygen from the lungs to the tissues **(Diez-Silva et al., 2010).**

- **White blood cells-** These cells also known as leukocytes or leucocytes, these are the cells of the immune system that are involved in protect the body against both infectious disease and foreign invaders. All white blood cells are formed and derived from multipotent cells in the bone marrow known as hematopoietic stem cells. Leukocytes are found all over the body, including the blood and lymphatic system **(Maton et al., 1997).**

- **Hemoglobin-** Hemoglobin is the protein molecule in red blood cells that carries oxygen from lungs to cells and return carbon dioxide from the tissues. It gives the red colour to the blood and rich in iron **(Berry et al., 2015).**
- **Platelets** – They also called thrombocytes (from Greek θρόμβος, "clot" and κύτος, "cell"), are a constituent of blood whose function (along with the coagulation factors) is to react to bleeding from blood vessel injury by clumping, thereby initiating a blood clot **(Laki, 1972).**

SIGNIFICANCE OF THE STUDY:

The study showed the effects of yoga. The findings of the study may help the individuals to compare the changes that occur in selected physical fitness, physiological and haemotological components before and after the yoga training programs. The study as such will create significant health awareness among people. The result of the study will provide the fundamental programs of yoga for school level students. The study will promoted research and growth in the field of yoga training. The study is very helpful to create the positive attitude towards Yoga Asana and Pranayama among students and all people of the society. The results of the study will give answer to the question, "Will Yoga Asana and Pranayama improve physical fitness, and increase physiological and haemotological health"? It is very useful to suggest the training program of Asana and Parayanama for a particular person. The study also motivates the new scholars to do research in fields of Yoga, Which is, now days very popular in every segment of the society.

SUMMARY OF THE CHAPTER:

This chapter presented and defined the research problem and importance of the study. Objectives of the study, hypotheses of the study, delimitations of the study, limitations of the study, significances of the study and definitions of the terms used in the study also have been explained in detail. This chapter presented an overview of the study. This chapter answers the entire questions that explained why this study was done, how was studied and what was studied. In the next chapter „Literature Review" presented an evaluation of previous researches related to the present study shows that there are gaps which will attempt to fill with the present study.

CHAPTER-II

REVIEW OF RELATED LITRATURE

Review of related literature is very essential requirement for proper preparation and implementation. The researcher necessitates obtaining latest information in relation to what has been considered and supposed in a meticulous area so that benefits can be derived from the work of their predecessors.

Investigation of related literature means to mark out, to know and to assess the earlier period as well as the modern literature of research concerned with the problem in hand for study. The main purpose of the study of allied literature is not assemblage but an analytical review of a variety of sources. It stimulates and encourages the particulars of the problems and enables the researcher to formulate hypothesis concerning their attainable solutions.

The research scholar has done his best and sincere efforts to locate the related literature concerned to the present study. Various researchers had tried to explain and present the effect of yoga on different variables at different levels. Different studies showed different results with some level of difference. Brief accounts of these studies are given in this chapter.

Madanmohan et al. (1992) determined effect of yoga training on visual and auditory reaction times (RTs), maximum expiratory pressure (MEP), maximum inspiratory pressure (MIP), 40 mmHg test, breath holding time after expiration (BHT exp), breath holding time after inspiration (BHT insp), and hand grip strength (HGS). For study purpose twenty seven (N=27) student volunteers were selected as the subjects. They were given yoga training for 12 weeks. The selected variables were tested before and after the yoga training. There was a significant ($P < 0.001$) decrease in visual RT (from 270.0 +/- 6.20 (SE) to 224.81 +/- 5.76 ms) as well as auditory Reaction Time (from 194.18 +/- 6.00 to 157.33 +/- 4.85 ms). MEP increased from 92.61 +/- 9.04 to 126.46 +/- 10.75 mmHg, while MIP increased from 72.23 +/- 6.45 to 90.92 +/- 6.03 mmHg, both these changes being statistically significant ($P < 0.05$). 40 mmHg test and HGS increased significantly ($P < 0.001$) from 36.57 +/- 2.04 to 53.36 +/- 3.95 s and 13.78 +/- 0.58 to 16.67 +/- 0.49 kg in that order. BHTexp increased from 32.15

+/- 1.41 to 44.53 +/- 3.78s ($P < 0.01$) and BHT insp increased from 63.69 +/- 5.38 to 89.07 +/- 9.61 s ($P < 0.05$). Results of the study showed that yoga training for 12 weeks creates significant diminution in visual and auditory reaction times and significant improvements in respiratory pressures, breath holding times and hand grip strength. The study results support that regular yoga training makes us physically and physiological strong.

Ray et al. (2001) observed the positive effect of yogic practices during training period on the young trainees. Total 54 young trainees were selected for the study. Their age ranged between 20-25 years. They were divided randomly in two groups i.e. yoga training group and control group. Yoga training group (23 males and 5 females) was administered yogic exercises for the first 5 months of the training while control group (21 males and 5 females) did not perform any exercises during this period. From the 6th to 10th month of training both the groups participated in the yoga practices. Physiological parameters like heart rate, blood pressure, oral temperature, skin temperature in resting condition, responses to maximal and submaximal exercise, body flexibility were selected and recorded. Psychological parameters like personality, learning, arithmetic and psychomotor ability and mental well being were also recorded for evaluation. Selected parameters were taken before and during the 5th and 10th month of training period. In starting there was relatively higher sympathetic activity in both the groups due to the new work/training environment and conditions. Later on at the 5th and 10th month, the experiment group (Yoga) had relatively lower sympathetic activity than the control group. The results of the study showed that there was considerable improvement in performance at submaximal level of exercise and in anaerobic threshold in the yoga group. Shoulder, hip, trunk and neck flexibility improved in the yoga group. There was significant improvement in various psychological variables like diminution in anxiety and depression and better mental function after participating in yoga training.

Tran et al. (2001) studied the effects of hatha yoga practice on the health-related aspects of Physical Fitness. To achieve the objectives of the study, ten (N=10) healthy, untrained volunteers (nine females and one male) were selected as the subjects. Their age ranged between 18-27 years. They were examined to determine the effects of hatha yoga training on the health-related aspects of physical fitness which were counting muscular strength, endurance, flexibility, cardiorespiratory fitness, body composition, and pulmonary function. Subjects were compulsory to join a minimum of two yoga training sessions per week for a total of 8 weeks. Each yoga session consisted of 10 minutes of pranayamas (breath-control exercises), 15 minutes of active warm-up exercises, 50 minutes of asanas (yoga postures), and 10 minutes of supine relaxation in savasana (corpse pose). The subjects were tested before and after the 8-week yoga training program. Isokinetic muscular strength for elbow extension, elbow flexion, and knee extension increased by 31%, 19%, and 28% ($p<0.05$), respectively, whereas isometric muscular endurance for knee flexion increased 57% ($p<0.01$). Ankle flexibility, shoulder elevation, trunk extension, and trunk flexion increased by 13% ($p<0.01$), 155% ($p<0.001$), 188% ($p<0.001$), and 14% ($p<0.05$), respectively. Absolute and relative maximal oxygen uptake increased by 7% and 6%, respectively ($p<0.01$). The findings of the study point out and support that regular hatha yoga practice produced improvements in the health-related aspects of physical fitness.

Kasiganesan et al. (2004) determined the effects of Hatha yoga and Omkar meditation on cardio respiratory performance, psychological profile, and melatonin secretion. To achieve the objectives of the study total thirty healthy men were selected for the study. Their age ranged in the age group of 25-35 years. They were volunteered for the study. They were randomly divided into two groups of 15 subjects in each group. Group 1 subjects served as controls group and performed body flexibility exercises for 40 minutes and slow running for 20 minutes during morning hours and played games for 60 minutes in evening hours daily for 3 months. Group 2 yoga training group subjects involved in selected yogic asanas (postures) for 45 minutes and pranayama for 15 minutes in the morning, whereas during the evening hours these subjects participated basic yogic postures for 15 minutes, pranayama for 15 minutes and meditation for 30 minutes daily, for 3 months. Orthostatic tolerance, heart rate, blood pressure, respiratory rate, dynamic lung function (such as forced vital capacity, forced expiratory volume in 1 second, forced expiratory volume percentage, peak expiratory flow rate, and maximum voluntary ventilation), and psychological profile were selected variables for the study. These were measured before and after 3 months of yogic practices. Serial blood samples were drawn at different time intervals to study effects of these yogic practices and Omkar meditation on melatonin levels. Yogic practices for 3 months resulted in an improvement in cardio respiratory performance and psychological profile. The results of the study also showed that the plasma melatonin significant increase after three months of yogic practices. The systolic blood pressure, diastolic blood pressure, mean arterial pressure, and orthostatic tolerance did not show any considerable relationship with plasma melatonin. However, the maximum night time melatonin levels in yoga group showed a significant correlation ($r = 0.71$, $p < 0.05$) with well-being score. These observations of the study showed that yogic practices can be used as psycho-physiologic stimuli to increase endogenous secretion of melatonin, which might be responsible for improved sense of well-being.

Clay et al. (2005) determined the metabolic and heart rate (HR) responses of hatha yoga. To achieve the purpose total 26 women were selected as the subjects. Their age ranged between 19-40 years. They performed 30-minute hatha yoga exercises of supine lying, sitting, and standing asanas. Subjects were followed the same videotaped sequences of hatha yoga asanas. Mean physiological variables responses were compared to the physiological responses of resting position on a chair and walking on a treadmill at 93.86 m.min (-1) [3.5 miles per hour (mph)] speed. During the 30-minute hatha yoga training, mean absolute oxygen consumption (Vo(2)), relative Vo(2), percentage of maximal oxygen consumption (%Vo(2)R), metabolic equivalents (METs), energy expenditure, HR, and percentage maximal heart rate (%MHR) were 0.45 L.min(-1), 7.59 ml.kg(-1).min(-1), 14.50%, 2.17 METs, 2.23 kcal.min(-1), 105.29 b.min(-1), and 56.89%, respectively. When compared to resting in a chair, hatha yoga required 114% greater O(2) (L.min(-1)), 111% greater O(2)(ml.kg(-1).min(-1)), 4,294% greater %Vo(2)R, 111% greater METs, 108% greater kcal.min(-1), 24% greater HR, and 24% greater %MHR. When compared to walking at 93.86 m.min(-1), hatha yoga required 54% lower O(2)(L.min(-1)), 53% lower O(2)(ml.kg(-1).min(-1)), 68% lower %Vo(2)R, 53% lower METs, 53% lower kcal.min(-1), 21% lower HR, and 21% lower %MHR. The hatha yoga routine in this study required 14.50% Vo(2)R, which can be considered a very low intensity and significantly lighter than 44.8% Vo(2)R for walking at 93.86 m.min(-1) (3.5 mph). The intensity of hatha yoga may be too low to construct a training stimulus for enhancing cardiovascular fitness. Although previous research suggests that hatha yoga is an acceptable form of physical activity for enhancing

Grabara and Szopa (2006) studied the hatha yoga exercises influence on health state of long term practitioners. Total 42 subjects were engaged (32 women and 10 men) at age range from 19-64 years. There were evaluated body height and mass, and next on their basis there was calculated relative body mass index (BMI). Moreover, there were carried out questionnaire interview concerning feeling of effects of hatha-yoga training on health state. Results of the study showed that hatha-yoga has ideal influence on health state of exercising persons. As measurable exercises effect respondents indicated significant improvements in body endurance and resistance, flexibility, muscles strengthening, stopping or diminution pain in different ailments, internal organs functioning improvement, body mass drop off, body slimming and metabolism regulating, energy, concentration and reflex increase, better sleep, mood, increase of own body awareness, movements smoothness, expansion of breath lasting time, gaining bigger harmony and relax in body, increasing of resistance on stress, distance to surrounding reality. However, no harmful effects were noticed of hatha yoga exercises system on organism. Results showed that hatha-yoga exercises are advantageous for everyone, in spite of of age or psychophysical conditions.

Edwards and Eldridge (2007) studied the effects of yoga on physiological indicators and perceived quality of Life. The purpose of the present study was to examine the effects of regular yoga exercises on weight, body composition, strength, flexibility, and perceived quality of life (via SF-36 questionnaire), as well as cardiovascular indicators such as heart rate, blood pressure, estimated aerobic capacity, and resting metabolic rate. Total forty two subjects (39 female, 3 male) were recruited as the subjects of the study. Each subject underwent to pre tests to determine baseline measures of the abovementioned factors. Then subjects were randomly assigned into experimental group and control group. Experimental group attended three (50-minute) flow-style yoga classes each week for 12 weeks. After end of the training program, all subjects were retested. Results of study showed that strength improved significantly ($p<.05$, $F=7.801$) as did flexibility ($p<.05$, $F=10.961$), and the mental component of the SF-36 health questionnaire ($p<.05$, $F=8.078$). Bicep curl strength increased considerably by .5 lbs for experimental group, while the control decreased strength by 3.86 pounds. Shoulder row strength better significantly by 4.64 pounds for experimental group, the control group decreased by 10.96 pounds. finally, experimental group improved leg press/back extension strength by 11.87 pounds while the control decreased by 13.30 pounds. Sit and reach flexibility increased by 3.18 inches, or 18%. The control group decreased sit and reach by .18 inches or a net change of-1%. Shoulder flexibility improved for the experimental group by 3.477 inches, while the shoulder flexibility for control decreased by 1.122 inches. The experimental group scored 47.53 pre-test to 54.46 post-test on the mental portion of the SF-36. Control group scored 47.81 pre-test and 50.96 post-test. Heart rate response data revealed subjects worked at 78% of estimated maximal heart rate. Study results verify that other findings in the literature concerning strength and flexibility gains with the regular practice of yoga. It also proves that yoga practice tends to considerably improve subjects' perception of quality of life. Current literature is unclear whether or not regular yoga practice has an aerobic benefit. Subjects' heart rate responses in this study were of adequate intensity to create aerobic improvement.

Hagins et al. (2007) evaluated that does practicing hatha yoga satisfy recommendations for intensity of physical activity which improves and maintains health and cardiovascular fitness. The objectives of this study were 1) to study whether yoga practice training meets the current recommendations for levels of physical activity mandatory to improve and maintain health and cardiovascular health; 2) to evaluate the reliability of metabolic costs of yoga across training sessions; 3) to compare the metabolic costs of yoga practice to those of treadmill walking. In this study to achieve the purpose, total 20 intermediate-to-advanced level yoga practitioners, age 31.4 +/- 8.3 years, performed an exercise schedule inside a human respiratory chamber (indirect calorimeter) while wearing heart rate monitors. The exercise routine made of 30 minutes of sitting, 56 minutes of beginner-level hatha yoga practices administered by video, and 10 minutes of treadmill walking at 3.2 and

4.8 kph each. The selected variables for the study were mean oxygen consumption (VO2), heart rate (HR), percentage predicted maximal heart rate (%MHR), metabolic equivalents (METs), and energy expenditure (kcal). Seven subjects repeated the whole procedure so that measurement reliability could be established. The results showed that Mean values across the entire yoga training programme for VO2, HR, %MHR, METs, and energy/min were 0.6 L/kg/min; 93.2 beats/min; 49.4%; 2.5; and 3.2 kcal/min; respectively. Results of the ICCs (2.1) for mean values across the whole yoga session for kcal, METs, and %MHR were 0.979 and 0.973, and 0.865, respectively. **Conclusion:** Metabolic costs of hatha yoga exercises averaged transversely the entire session showed low levels of physical activity, are similar to walking on a treadmill at 3.2 kph, and do not meet recommendations for levels of physical activity for improving or maintaining health or cardiovascular fitness. Yoga practice incorporating sun salutation postures more than the minimum bout of 10 minutes may contribute some portion of sufficiently intense physical activity to get better cardio-respiratory fitness in unfit or inactive persons. The measurement of energy expenditure across yoga sessions is highly reliable.

Ulger et al. (2007) examined the effects of Hatha yoga training on flexibility and balance of healthy women. To conduct this study total 25 volunteer women were selected. The age of the subjects ranged between 30-45 years. They did not have any health problems to attend this study. Demographic characteristics, flexibility and balance consideration tests were done before the hatha yoga training. The subjects participated in the hatha yoga training sessions for 8 weeks for one hour, 2 times in a week. Their assessments were repeated when yoga training sessions were completed. Results of the study: There was no significant difference between the groups in regards to demographic characteristics in pre test. There were significant improvements in flexibility values of all subjects between pre and post yoga sessions ($p<0.05$). A significant difference was found between pre and post yoga exercises training during balance test with closed eyes on right and left extremities correspondingly ($p<0.05$). The results of this study showed that it is possible to use yoga based exercises in healthy subjects for preventive means. Hatha yoga training improved flexibility and balance considerably. So it is proved that yoga training have positive effects on physical fitness related variables.

Madanmohan et al. (2008) studied that whether yoga training of six weeks duration modulates sweating response to dynamic exercise and improves respiratory pressures, handgrip strength and handgrip endurance. Total 46 healthy subjects (30 males and 16 females, age ranged between 17-20 years) were selected. They were divided in two groups. 23 motivated subjects (15 male and 8 female) were undergone yoga training and the remaining 23 subjects treated as the control group. Weight loss following Harvard step test (an index of sweat loss), maximum inspiratory pressure, maximum expiratory pressure, 40 mm endurance, handgrip strength and handgrip endurance were selected variables which were measured before and after the six weeks training period. In the yoga group, weight loss in response to Harvard step test was 64 +/- 30 g after yoga training as compared to 161 +/- 133 g before the training and the difference was significant (n = 15 male subjects, P < 0.0001). In contrast, weight loss following step test was not considerably changed in the control group at the end of the study period. Yoga training produced a marked improvement in respiratory pressures and endurance in 40 mm Hg test in both male and female subjects (P < 0.05 for all comparisons). In conclusion, the present study presents attenuation of the sweating response to step test by yoga training. Further, yoga training of six weeks can produce significant improvements in respiratory muscle strength and endurance.

Bal and Kaur (2009) investigated the effects of selected Asanas in hatha yoga on agility and flexibility level. Total thirty (N=30) male students from D.A.V. institute of engineering and technology, Jalandhar (Punjab), India were selected as the subjects. Random group design method was used for selection of the subjects. All subjects age ranged between 18-25 years. They were divided into two groups. Group –A (N=15) treated as an experimental group and Group-B acts a control group. To monitor the quality of the subjects "Hexagonal obstacle test" was used where as to test flexibility „sit and reach test was used. A six weeks yoga asana training programme was subjected to experimental group. The training programme includes swastikasna, mayurasana, matsyendrasana, paschimottanasana and gomukhasana. The time of one training session was 90 minutes. Pre and post test were conducted to know the effects of training. The difference in the mean of each group for selected variables were tested for the significance of difference by „t"test. The level of significance was set at 0.05. The results of the study showed that the mean of flexibility of pre test of experimental group was 47.86 and post test mean was 50.20. whereas for control group the mean of flexibility for pre and post test were 46.66 and 46.800 respectively. The „t"value in case of experimental group was 8.122 and for control group it was 0.414. Since cal. „t"(=8.122) > tab „t"0.05 (=2.145). So it showed that six weeks of yogasana training showed significant improvement in flexibility. For agility the experimental group mean for pre test was 14.70 and post test mean was 13.42 whereas for control group mean for pre test was 15.41 and for post test was 15.03. The „t"value in case of experimental group was -7.3 and for control group it was -5.389. (= -7.3) > 0.05. So six weeks yogasana training also showed significant improvement in agility.

Javnbakht et al. (2009) determined the influence of yoga in relieving symptoms of depression and anxiety in women who were referred to a yoga clinic. In the study a convenience sample of women were involved who were referred to a yoga clinic from July 2006 to July 2007. All new cases were evaluated on admission using a personal information questionnaire well as Beck and Spielberger tests. Subjects of the study were randomly assigned into the experimental and the control group. The experimental group (n=34) participated for two days in a week. One yoga session was 90 minutes of duration for two months. The control group (n=31) was assigned to a waiting list and did not receive yoga. Both groups were evaluated again after the two-month of yoga training period. The average prevalence of depression in the experimental group pre and post Yoga intervention was 12.82+/-7.9 and 10.79+/-6.04 respectively. It was a statistically inconsequential reduction (p=0.13). However, when the experimental group was compared to the control group, subjects who participated in yoga classes showed a significant decrease in state anxiety (p=0.03) and trait anxiety (p<0.001). Participation in a two-month yoga training sessions can lead to significant decrease in perceived levels of anxiety in women who suffer from anxiety disorders. The results of the study suggest that yoga can be considered as a complementary therapy and also used as an alternative method for medical therapy in the treatment of anxiety disorders.

Heo et al. (2010) examined the effects of yoga training program on physical fitness, depression and quality of life of elderly women in rural area. This study was conducted on experimental and control group pre test –post test design. A total of 40 elderly women (experimental group =20) and control group =20) were selected as subjects from H-gun, G-Province. The experimental group participated in a 12 weeks yoga program. In physical fitness, the experimental group taking yoga program reported significant improvements in balance and flexibility than that in the control group, but the differences in strength and aerobic endurance were not considerably improved. The experimental group of the study showed significant decrease in the depression. In quality of life, Elderly women taking yoga program had significant increase in physical component summary compared to control group, but differences in mental component summary was not significant. A yoga program may be very useful for elderly women in rural area to improve their balance, flexibility, to reduce depression and improve physical quality of life.

Mazumdar and Suryavanshi (2010) analysed the effect of Ujjayi and Bhastrika Pranayama on selected physiological variables. Total 60 physically challenged male students were randomly selected as the subjects from Amar jyoti public school and Roshni Rehabilitation Centre, Gwalior. Further they were divided into two groups: the experimental group and the control group. The experimental group was assigned for Ujjayi and Bhastrika Pranayama for 5 days in a week for the period of 6 weeks. The training was given in the morning. Four physiological variables vital capacity, positive breath holding time, resting pulse rate and blood pressure were selected for the study. Pre- and post-test data on selected physiological variables were measured before and after completion of 6 weeks pranayama training of experimental group. The control group did not participate in any special training programme. The criterion method for measuring vital capacity was evaluated with Recorder and Medicare Systems Spirometer (Helios 401) in litres, breath holding and resting pulse rate was measured with the help of stopwatch, and blood pressure was measured by sphygmomanometer and stethoscope. Paired „t"test statistical technique was used to analyse the recorded raw data, and the mean difference between the pre -test and post-test scores each of the criterion variables of the groups. The level of significance was fixed at 0.05 level. From the results of the study it was observed that „t" ratio was not significant in case of resting pulse rate and diastolic blood pressure. However in case of vital capacity and breath holding time t- ratio was significantly improved.

Coelho et al. (2011) determined that whether the regular practice of Hatha Yoga could have impacts on quality of life in a group of healthy women. This study was a transversal controlled study. For this study total 25 women were selected as the subjects of the study. Their age ranged between 20-59 years. They were divided into two groups: Yoga Group (N=13) and the control group (N=12). Yoga group participated in six months Hatha yoga practices programme and control group did not attend any specific exercises program. The quality of life of healthy women was assessed through the SF-36 questionnaire. The statistical measures used for results of the study were independent„t"-test and the Mann-Whitney tests. The YOGA group showed higher scores in the "body pain" domain and in the general physical score (p < 0,05). It can be concluded that the regular practice of Hatha Yoga exercises has positively and significantly influenced some aspects of the quality of life.

Gaurav (2011) determined the effects of hatha yoga exercises on health related physical fitness variables including muscular Strength, Agility, Power, Speed and Cardiovascular Endurance. To achieve the objectives of the study total thirty male students selected randomly from Department of Physical Education Guru Nanak Dev University, Amritsar (Punjab, India). The age of the subjects ranged between 18 –24 years. They were volunteered to participate in the study. Subjects were assigned into two groups: A (experimental: N-15) and B (control: N-15). The students from Group A were subjected to 8-weeks hatha yoga training programme. Each yoga training assembly consisted of 10 minutes of pranayamas , 15 minutes of active warm-up exercises, 40 minutes of asanas and 5 minutes of supine relaxation in savasana. The subjects were tested pre and post of the 8-week yoga training program. Statistically t-test was used to assess the between-group differences for dependent data to assess the Post-Pre differences. Results revealed that the health related physical fitness variables including muscular Strength, Agility, Power (p<0.01) and Speed (p<0.05) considerably improved in experimental yoga group as compared to control group. On the other hand experimental group showed non-significant improvement in cardiovascular endurance. These findings of the study verify that regular hatha yoga exercises can bring out improvements in the health-related variables of physical fitness and may contribute to enhance our health status and wellness.

Grabara and Szopa (2011) assessed the effects of hatha yoga exercises on the shaping of the antero-posterior spinal curvature in first-year students of the University of Physical Education in Katowice. They participated in hatha yoga classes. Total 72 women and 46 men were selected for the study. Hatha yoga training sessions were held one time in a week for 90 minutes for the period of 15 weeks. Measurements of the subjects' spines were performed twice, first before the start of the hatha yoga trainings and then after all the training classes were ended. The subjects were divided into three groups, the first group composed of all the participants in the study, the second group of subjects whom attended the yoga classes and practiced hatha yoga in their free time, whereas the third group was composed of subjects for whom hatha yoga training was their only form of physical exercise. The inclination of the anteroposterior curvature of the spine, i.e. the thoracic kyphosis and lumbar lordosis angles, were measured with a Rippstein plurimeter. The results of the study showed that after 15 weeks of yoga, a decrease in the thoracic kyphosis angle (ThKA) and lumbar lordosis angle (LLA) occurred in most of the students. Differences between the values of these angles before/after yoga were statistically considerable in women ($p < 0.001$), whereas in men, only a decrease of the thoracic kyphosis angle was statistically significant ($p < 0.001$). After finishing the hatha yoga classes, the majority of subjects (50-62%) were found to have correct angular standards of the thoracic kyphosis and lumbar lordosis when compared to the dimensions taken before the start of classes (40-45%). Conclusion of the study: An assessment on the shaping of the anteroposterior curvature of the spine finds that hatha yoga trainings have a positive and significantly impact on one's body posture in the sagittal plane.

Singh et al. (2011) studied the effects of 6-weeks yoga asana training on agility and muscular strength in sportsmen. To achieve the purpose of the study thirty male sports persons were randomly selected from department of physical education, Guru Nanak Dev University, Amritsar (Punjab, India). Their age ranged from 18 – 24 years. They were volunteered to participate in the study. They were randomly divided into two groups: Y (experimental N=15) and C (control N=15). The subjects from Group Y were assigned to a 6-weeks yoga asana training programme. Pre and post test were conducted to collect the data. For results of the study„t" test was used to assess the between-group differences for dependent data to assess the Post-Pre differences. The level of $p \leq 0.01$ was fixed for significant. The agility and muscular strength significantly increased in Group Y compared with the control group. The results of the study recommended yoga asana training to improve agility and muscular strength and it does also contribute to enhance sports performance.

Yokesh (2012) studied the impact of yogic practice and aerobic exercise on selected Physical and physiological variables among overweight school boys. To achieve the objectives, forty five overweight school boys students from various schools in Tiruchirappalli district were randomly selected. Their age ranged between 14 and 17 years. The selected students were randomly divided into three equal groups of 15 each, namely yogic exercise group (group A), Aerobic exercise group (group B) and control group (group C). The experimental group A participated in yogic training and group B in aerobic exercise. They participated in their respective trainings five days a week for 12 weeks. The control group (group C) maintained their daily routine activities and no specific training was given. Physical parameter namely flexibility and physiological variable breath holding time were chosen as the variables for the study. The subjects of the three groups were evaluated using standardized tests and procedures on selected physical and physiological variables. The data was collected before and after the training period. The following test items namely sit and reach and breath holding time were used to collect relevant data. The collected data were analyzed statistically with analysis of Covariance (ANCOVA) to find out the pre and post training performances to compare the significant difference between the adjusted final means and better group from all. The results showed that yogic exercise and aerobics exercise produced considerable improvement on flexibility and breathe holding time compared to control group.

Gaur et al. (2013) evaluated the effect of yoga training on cardio-respiratory functions of normal young volunteers. To achieve the objectives of the study 15 healthy male (18-20 years) were selected. They were given 10 weeks yoga training that included asanas and pranayams. Blood pressure, heart rate and respiratory parameters were tested prior and post of 10 week yoga training programme. Results of the study: Yoga training produced a significant decrease in resting blood pressure, heart rate and rate-pressure product, indicating a reduction in load on the heart. These results support and showed that yoga has a cardio-protective role. Yoga training produced a significant increase in respiratory pressures and 40 mmHg endurance indicative of that yoga exercise increases the strength of expiratory as well as inspiratory muscles and cardio-respiratory endurance. Breath holding time also improves significantly after yoga training. Conclusion: The present study result has shown that 10 week yoga training improves cardio-respiratory functions in normal young volunteers.

Huang et al. (2013) studied the comparative effectiveness of a single 90-minute Hatha yoga class and an 8-week, 90-minute-class-per-week course. To achieve the objectives of the study a quasi experimental design was used. Total 63 female community residents in New Taipei City aged 40-60 years were selected as the subjects. They were randomly divided into an experimental group (n = 30) and a control group (n = 33). The experimental group participated in the 8-weeks Hatha yoga training course. The control group received no specific training. The Perceived Stress Scale (PSS) and heart rate variability (HRV) determined stress reduction effectiveness. Chi-square, independent t test, paired t test, and generalized estimating equations were used as the statistical techniques for data analysis of the study. Results of the study showed that after a single 90-minute hatha yoga training class, experimental group PSS scores were notably decreased than those of the control group ($p = .001$). Although experimental group HRV (low-frequency norm and high-frequency norm) had increased but these changes were not statistically significant ($p = .059$). PSS scores for the single 90-minute class and 8-week course did not considerably different to each other ($p = .157$) and HRV of statistics is significant ($p = .005$). Generalized estimating equations analyzed changes in the effectiveness over time of stress lessening (HRV and PSS) after the Hatha yoga training program. Results showed the post hatha yoga training HRV and PSS of the experimental group less significantly ($p < .001$) more than the control group. Findings of the study support that regular, long-term practice of Hatha yoga provides clear and significant health benefits for subjects. Participation in a single 90-minute Hatha yoga class can notably decrease perceived stress. Regularly practising hatha yoga for a long period can reduce perceived stress even more considerably.

Murugavel and Laxmi (2013) determined the effects of asana and core training on breath holding time, vo2 max and resting pulse rate level of middle aged working women. The sample for the study consisted of sixty middle aged women. Their age ranged between 35-50 years. They were divided into two groups, 1.The control group and the experimental group. The control group was not given any specific training treatment and the experimental group was given asana and core training programme. They participated in asana and core training for five days per week for a period of 8 weeks. All the subjects were subjected to measure for selected variables for pre and post test. Physiological variables of breath holding time, vo 2 max and resting pulse rate level. The data collected from the subjects were statistically analyzed with the help of „t" ratio to find out significant difference among experimental group and control group and physiological variables if any. The results of the study indicate that eight weeks of asana and core training programme produced significant improvement in breath holding time, vo2 max and resting pulse rate.

Subramani (2013) determined the effect of yoga asanas with pranayama practices on resilience and assertiveness among women students. To achieve the objectives of this study, total 24 women students were randomly selected from women's hostel, Manonmaniam Sundaranar University, Tirunelveli, Tamilnadu, India as the subjects of the study. Their age ranged between 23 to 28 years. The selected students were randomly divided into two equal Groups such as Group 'A' yoga asanas with pranayama exercises (n=12) and Group 'B' acted as control group (n=12). Group 'A' participated in yoga asanas with pranayama training program for five days per week and each session lasted for an hour for six weeks. Control group did not undergo any specific training but they participated in regular activities. The selected variables namely resilience and assertiveness were measured by the standardized questionnaire. The data was collected prior and after of 6 weeks of training. The pre and post-test scores were statistically evaluated by the dependent 't' test and Analysis of Co-

Variance (ANCOVA) for selected variable. The results of the study showed that the yoga asanas with pranayama training group had shown significantly improvement in resilience and assertiveness. The Control group had not shown any significant improvement on any of the selected variable such as Resilience and Assertiveness.

Whiddon and Bazini (2013) evaluated the effects of Hatha yoga on depression in adults. It was believed that regular practice of yoga restores the good mental and physical health. Methods of study: to archive the purpose of the study true experimental method was used. Twenty-six adults from mid-sized, urban city in Central Florida were selected as the subjects of the study. They suffered from mild, moderate, to severe depression. The subjects were divided in the experimental and the control-group. Subjects in the experimental group practiced Hatha yoga for one and a half hours, three times in a week, for eight weeks. Pre test-post test design was used. Subjects in the control group were on a wait list. The Beck Depression Inventory-II was used as a pre test and post test compute and an independent sample t-test was used to analyse the data of the study. Results: The results of the study showed that the BDI-II depression scores for the individuals in the experimental group were significantly decreased than the control group. Conclusions: The study results support previous research that Hatha yoga is feasible and effective for treatment for reducing depressive symptoms.

Hainsworth et al. (2014) examined whether Hatha yoga would improve overall, physical and psychosocial functioning in youth with severe obesity. They also wanted to determine whether participants would increase the vigour of, and time spent in, physical activity. To achieve the objectives of the study total 16 youth with severe obesity were selected. This study utilized a pre-test/post-test design. Sixteen youth with severe obesity completed an 8 week Hatha yoga intervention involving fifteen, 60-minute classes. Physical and psychosocial functioning, fitness and state-anxiety were assessed at baseline and post-intervention; parents completed proxy-reports of physical and psychosocial functioning at both time points. To assess physical activity, participants wore an Actical Accelerometer for 7 days pre and post-yoga. Results: considerable improvements were found in: Overall, Physical and Psychosocial functioning back and hamstring flexibility, and state-anxiety. Changes in the proportion of time spent in both light and modest levels of physical activity were marginally significant. Although 3 tests of fitness, and time spent in physical activity did not improve significantly, trends were in the expected direction. Conclusions: Youth with severe obesity may advantage from a Hatha yoga intervention. Yoga may also offer a way to engage in physical activity that is not precluded by bodily pain.

Prado et al. (2014) studied the effects of a hatha yoga training program on body balance in young adults. To achieve the objectives of the study used a controlled, nonrandomized design. The experimental group of the study underwent a 5-month hatha yoga training program and were then compared with the control group that had no specific training program. A convenience sample of 34 out of 40 men age ranged between 25-55 years old (34.0 ± 0.9) were selected for this study. They were randomly divided into two groups: Experimental group and control group. Subjects in the experimental group participated in 60 min sessions of hatha yoga training. The training was conducted three times in a week for 5 months. Evaluation of postural control was by measuring the limit of stability and velocity of oscillation (VOS) in three conditions of the balance rehabilitation unit (BRU) and through field procedures (four position, plane, flamingo, hopscotch, and dynamic test). In the results of the study observed differences ($P < 0.05$) in post tests scores between the groups regardless of BRU parameters and field procedures (except for flamingo) even after adjusting for prior to training test scores, suggesting that these changes were created by hatha yoga exercises. The partial eta squared on BRU parameters ranged from 0.78 (VOS1)-0.97 (COP2), and from 0.00 (flamingo)-0.94 (four position) for the field procedures. Conclusions: Our results provide significant support that postural control in healthy young adults can be improved considerably through practising hatha yoga.

Sieverdes et al. (2014) determined the effects of Hatha yoga on blood pressure, salivary α-amylase, and cortisol function among normotensive and prehypertensive youth. Total thirty-one (N=31) seventh graders were randomly selected for the study and divided into two groups: Hatha yoga group and attention control group. They were assigned to a Hatha yoga program (HYP) and attention control (AC) music or art class respectively. Prior to training and after 3-month training data collection were included. Resting BP; overnight urine samples; and saliva collected at bedtime, upon awakening, and at 30 and 60 minutes after awakening for α-amylase and cortisol were measured. Twenty-eight (14 in the HYP group and 14 in the AC group) students were assessed both before and after the intervention. BP changes from pre- to post-intervention were -3.0/-2.0 mmHg for the HYP group and -0.07/-0.79 mmHg for the AC group (p=0.30 and 0.57, respectively). Changes in systolic blood pressure (SBP) / diastolic blood pressure (DBP) for the prehypertensive (75th-94th percentiles for SBP) subgroup analyses were -10.75/-8.25 mmHg for the Hatha yoga training group (n=4) versus 1.8/1.0 mmHg for the AC group (n=5) (p for SBP=0.02; p for DBP=0.09). There were no statistically significant group differences noticed with changes in SNS or HPA awakening curves (area under curve for α-amylase and cortisol, respectively) and a small to modest effect was seen favouring a diminution of α-amylase activation for the Hatha Yoga Programme group (Cohen d=0.34; prehypertensive d=0.20). **Conclusions:** A school level students-based Hatha yoga program showed potential to decrease resting BP, particularly among prehypertensive youth. Reduced SNS drive may be an core neuro hormonal pathway beneficially affected by the program. A large-scale efficacy/usefulness randomized clinical trial is needed.

Kumar (2015) organised a study to find out the effect of Asanas, Pranayama and combined practices on selected Physical, Psychological, Physiological and Hematological Variables among Degree College Students. In the present study, total sixty students were selected by random sampling from S.S.R Government College, Andhra Pradesh as the subjects. The subjects selected for the study were divided randomly into four equal groups called Experimental Group – I (Asanas group), Experimental Group - II (Pranayama group), Experimental Group - III Combined practices (Asanas and Pranayama group) and Group IV - Control group and their age ranged from 19 to 25 years. Further the role of the students during the training and the testing process was also explained to them in detail. Twelve weeks of Asanas, Pranayama, and Combined training (Asanas and Pranayama) were given to the experimental groups. The control group was not allowed to participate in any of the training programmes, except in their routine physical education programmes. The experimental groups participated in the training programme as per the training schedule made ready by the researcher. The training programme was held six days in a week for 12 weeks. The training was conducted by a qualified yoga trainer and was personally supervised by the investigator. The Physical Variables used in the present study were agility, flexibility and cardiovascular endurance. The Psychological variables were anxiety, Stress and Aggression. The Physiological Variables used were Resting Pulse Rate, Mean arterial Blood Pressure and Vital Capacity. The Hematological variables were Red Blood Cell, White Blood Cell and Hemoglobin. All the subjects were motivated to give relevant data and co-operate to complete the psychological questionnaire. The data obtained were analyzed by Analysis of Covariance (ANCOVA) to assess the significant difference among the groups between the pre test and post test on physical, psychological physiological and hematological variables The results of the study showed that the physical variables Agility, Flexibility and Cardiovascular endurance were significantly improved due to Twelve weeks of Asanas (Experimental Group - I), Pranayama (Experimental Group - II) and Combined Training (Asanas and Pranayama) (Experimental Group - III) among Degree college students comparing to the control group. The Psychological Variables Stress, Anxiety and Aggression were significantly altered (decrease) due to Twelve weeks of Asanas Pranayama and Combined Training (Asanas and Pranayama) among Degree college students. The Physiological variables Pulse rate and Mean arterial blood pressure were significantly decreased and Vital Capacity was significantly improved in all experimental groups due to twelve weeks of yoga trainings. The Hematological variable Hemoglobin, RBC and WBC were showed significantly improvements due to yoga trainings in all experimental groups. Finally the post hoc analysis of the results showed that Combined (Asanas and Pranayama, Group-III) was slightly more effective than Asanas(Group - I) and Pranayama (Group - II) in Agility, Flexibility, Cardiovascular Endurance, Anxiety, Aggression, Stress, Pulse Rate, Mean Arterial Blood pressure, Vital Capacity, Hemoglobin, Red Blood Cell and White Blood Cell.

Mohanty et al. (2015) studied that yoga practice increases minimum muscular fitness in children with visual impairment. Muscle strength is a very important constituent for balance, gait and functional mobility for children with visual impairment. Yoga has been frequently used to improve physical and mental fitness in children. This study designed to know the effect of 16 weeks yoga training on muscular fitness in children with visual impairment. To achieve the objectives of the study total eighty subjects were selected. They were divided in to two groups (41 subjects for yoga group and 39 subjects for control group). visual impairment students of both genders aged 9-16 years ranged on age, gender and degree of blindness were assessed at pre, mid (after 8 weeks) and post (after 16 weeks) yoga intervention using the Kraus-Weber test. The results of the study showed that the percentage of students passed in the test: yoga group were 12.2%, 43.9% and 68.3% whereas percentages in the control group were 23.1%, 30.8% and 30.8% in pre, mid, and post tests respectively. Mc Nemar test showed considerable improvements between pre and mid, mid and post in the yoga group while those parameters did not significantly improved in the control group. Yoga treatment seemed to have significant benefits for the children's muscular fitness. Conclusion: The study suggests that yoga has substantial benefits for improvement of fitness level in children with visual impairment and may be recommended as an effective, substitute, inexpensive low risk training activity option for them.

Rachiwong et al. (2015) studied the effects of modified hatha yoga in industrial rehabilitation on physical fitness and stress of injured workers. Total 18 male and female injured workers, age ranged between 18 to 55 years, participated in this study. They were divided into two groups. Groups-1 – an additive hatha yoga training to routine industrial rehabilitation programme group (HYG: n= 9) and a control group with no specific yoga training (CG: n= 9). A specific yoga protocol was designed for training group by two certified yoga instructors and conducted by for 1 hour, three times in a week for 8 weeks. Physical fitness variables included flexibility, of lower back and hamstrings, hand grip strength and lungs capacity. Score of sensitivity to stress was also evaluated at time of recruitment of subjects and after 8 weeks of intervention. The results of the study showed that the value of all fitness variables and stress score were not significantly different between the hatha yoga group and control group at pre test level. Post test results showed significant improvements in hatha yoga training group in flexibility, hand grip strength and vital capacity. On the other hand there was no significant change in control group. No significant change occurred in stress scores as a result of hatha yoga training.

Dharmalingam (2016) evaluated the effect of asana and pranayama practices on selected physical and physiological variables of college men. To achieve the purpose of the study, total 30 college men were selected from Sri Ramakrishna Vidyalaya College of arts and science, periyanaickenpalayam, Coimbatore as the subjects of the study. The age of the selected students were ranged between 17-21 years. Flexibility and balance were taken as a physical fitness variable and resting heart rate, cardiovascular endurance and vital capacity were taken as physiological variables for the study. The selected subjects participated in the 12 weeks of asana and pranayama training program, the pre and post-test were taken from the subjects before and after the 12 weeks of yoga training sessions. The paired sample T test was used to find out the significant difference between the pairs. From the statistical result it was concluded that the asana and pranayama exercises will significantly improve the physical fitness and physiological variables namely flexibility, balance, resting heart rate, cardio respiratory endurance and vital capacity in the level of 0.05 level of significance.

Bedekar and Hande (2017) concluded the effect of yoga on Cardio Respiratory endurance, Body Composition, Flexibility and Muscular strength of females. To achieve the purpose of the study thirty female participants were selected from Pravara Institute of Medical Science, Loni as the subjects of the study. Their age ranged from 18 to 25 years. The present study was organised to find out the effect of intervention of yoga on health related physical fitness components. Cardio respiratory endurance, Body composition (Body Mass Index), Flexibility and Muscular strength were selected as variables of the study. These all were evaluated before and after four weeks of yoga training. The data obtained was analyzed using paired „t" test. Significance level was fixed at $P < 0.0001$. Result of the study showed that: There was a significant improvement in the Cardio respiratory endurance ($p=0.0001$), Body Mass Index ($p=0.0001$), Flexibility ($p=0.0001$), and Muscular strength ($p=0.0001$) after yoga training program for four weeks when compared to that before yoga. Conclusion: Yoga is very useful for both physical and psychological aspects of the body through a series of low impact exercises, the results concluded that four weeks of Yoga training through yoga asana was found to be effective in bringing about considerable improvement in respect to Cardio respiratory endurance, Body Composition, Flexibility and Muscular strength.

Bhavanani et al. (2017) studied the effects of short term asana and pranayama training on reaction time. Many studies showed the long and short term effects of Yoga training on reaction time (RT), but very few studies have evaluated differential effects of asana and Pranayama trainings. The present study was done to elucidate effects of such differential training on reaction time (RT) in health professions students attending Yoga asana and pranayama training. Total 134 healthy young adults studying BSc Nursing at KGNC were selected for the study. 89 subjects from 1st year were randomly divided into two groups. 44 subjects of them received one week of training in asana while 45 subjects received parallel training in pranayama. 45 control subjects were recruited from 2nd year BSc Nursing and they didn"t receive any Yoga training. Auditory and visual reaction time (ART and VRT) were measured prior and post of the one week study period. (ANOVA) Post hoc testing was done by Dunn"s Multiple Comparisons Test. P values of less than 0.05 were taken to be indicating statistically significant differences and merely paired t tests done for intra group comparison. Results of the study showed that both asana and pranayama training resulted in significant ($p<0.001$) shortening of ART and VRT, while ART was significantly ($p<0.05$) prolonged in controls with no significant change in VRT. Intergroup comparisons showed that these changes were more pronounced following pranayama training especially with regard to VRT. Conclusion: The present study showed that even a short term, one week training in yoga asana and pranayama can shorten Reaction time and that this is more pronounced in case of pranayama training. These changes may be attributed to enhanced central processing ability resulting from better sense of perception, sensitivity, alertness and awareness occurring as a result of Yoga exercises. As pranayama training tends to be more introspectional (with eyes closed), this may have better effects than asana where awareness is more externalized in novices.

Chauhan et al. (2017) evaluated the effect of 1-month yoga practice on body mass index (BMI), and blood pressure (BP). The present study was conducted to find out the effect of yoga practice on 64 participants (age 53.6 ± 13.1 years) (experimental group) whereas the results were compared with 26 healthy volunteers (control group). The study examined the effects of yoga on physiological parameters in a 1-month pilot study. Most of the participants were beginners and practiced yoga for 1 hr. daily in the morning for 1 month. BMI and BP (systolic and diastolic) were studied before and after 1 month of yoga practice. **Results:** Yoga practice causes decreased BMI (26.4 ± 2.5-25.22 ± 2.4), systolic BP (136.9 ± 22.18 mmHg to 133 ± 21.38 mmHg), and diastolic BP (84.7 ± 6.5 mmHg to 82.34 ± 7.6 mmHg). On the other hand, no significant changes were observed in BMI and BP of control group. **Conclusion:** This study concludes that yoga practice has potential to control BMI and BP without taking any medication.

Kim and Ju (2017) examined the effects of the application of elderly-customized hatha yoga on the vascular inflammation factors of elderly women. The study was conducted with 14 elderly women, between 70 and 80 years old. They were divided into an elderly-customized hatha yoga group (n=7) and a control group (n=7). The hatha yoga group participated in a hatha yoga program designed to be elderly-friendly for 10 weeks. At the end of the yoga training program, the vascular inflammation parameters were measured, including the albumin, white blood cell count, fibrinogen, high sensitivity C-reactive protein (hs-CRP), and erythrocyte sedimentation rate (ESR). Results of the study showed that in the hatha yoga training group, the albumin improved significantly after the participation in training, when compared to the level before the treatment, while the fibrinogen, hs-CRP, and ESR decreased significantly. In the control group, the vascular inflammation factors level pre and post tests score was not significantly changed. Based on the results of this study, it is demonstrate that the application of elderly-customized hatha yoga produced positive changes in the vascular inflammation factors of elderly women.

Papp et al. (2017) determined the effects and feasibility of hatha yoga training program (HYP) compared to a conventional training program (CTP) on functional capacity, lung function and quality of life in patients with obstructive pulmonary diseases. The design of the study was based on randomized clinical trial study. The study was planned at the Karolinska University Hospital, Stockholm, among outpatients. To achieve the purposes total thirty-six (24 women and 12 men, median age =64, age range: 40-84 years) patients with obstructive pulmonary disease were selected. They were randomly divided into two groups: HYP Group (N.=19) and CTP Group (N.=17). Both hatha yoga group and conventional training group involved in a 12-weeks program with a 6-month follow-up. Functional capacity (using the 6-Minute Walk Test), lung function (spirometry), respiratory muscle strength (respiratory pressure meter), oxygen saturation (SpO2), breathlessness (Borg), respiratory rate (f) and disease-specific quality of life (CRQ) were selected as the variables of the study. These variables were calculated at baseline, at 12 weeks and at a 6-month follow-up. The results of the study showed that testing for interactions (group x time) with ANOVAs showed considerable effects on the CRQ fatigue (P=0.04) and emotional (P=0.02) domains, with increase in the conventional training group after the 12-week intervention (P=0.02 and 0.01, respectively) but not significant in the hatha yoga group. No between group effects emerged, however, within each group, considerable improvements emerged for the six-minute walk distance (6MWD) after 12-week intervention (HY: mean difference 32.6 m; CI: 10.1-55.1, P=0.014; CTP: mean difference 42.4 m; CI: 17.9-67.0, P=0.006). Within-group enhancements in CRQ appeared in both groups. Within the hatha yoga group, f decreased and SpO2 increased. Improved effects after follow-up emerged only for the conventional training group for diastolic blood pressure (P=0.05) and CRQ emotional and fatigue domain (P=0.01). **Conclusions:** There were no intergroup differences. After 12 weeks, 6MWD improved significantly within both groups. Within the hatha yoga group, improvements in the CRQ mastery domain, f and SpO2 emerged. Within the conventional training group, there were improvements in lung function consideration forced vital capacity, respiratory muscle strength and all CRQ-domains. The CTP also exhibited effects on CRQ after the 6months follow-up.

Rejinadevi and Ramesh (2017) determined the effect of yogic practices on selected physiological variables among basketball players. To achieve purpose of the study forty men basketball players were randomly selected as subjects from S.V.N College and Arul Anandar College, Madurai, Tamilnadu. Their age ranged from 18 to 25 years. The selected players were divided in to two groups of twenty players each. Group I acted as a Yogic practices group and Group II acted as a control group. The experimental group participated in Yoga practices training programme for twelve weeks duration in addition to their regular professional activities of the college as per the core curriculum. The control group did not participate in any training programme other than their daily routine actions. The criterion measures systolic blood pressure and diastolic blood pressure was evaluated by sphygmomanometer. The two groups were statistically analysed by using analysis of covariance (ANCOVA) at 0.05 level of significance. The result of the study reveals that there was a significant improvement in the experimental group on selected variables when compared to the control group after the completion of twelve weeks of yogic practices.

Shiraishi et al. (2017) evaluated the effects of a 12-week systematized yoga intervention on health-related physical fitness. Body mass, body mass index (BMI), waist circumference (WC), relative body fat, abdominal endurance, upper body endurance, hamstring flexibility, and cardio respiratory fitness were selected as dependent variables of the study. The study was performed at University of Brasília, Faculty of Physical Education, Distrito Federal, Brazil. To achieve the purpose of the study twenty-five young healthy yoga novices (22.36 ± 2.40 years), both gender, volunteeres were selected to participate in this study. The yoga intervention was based on 50 minutes yoga class, twice a week for 12 weeks, involving physical poses, meditation, and relaxation. Measurements of selected variables were performed one week prior to and one week after the yoga training completed. Collecting data included age, gender, height, body mass, body fat estimates and physical fitness tests of the subjects. Body fat percentage was evaluated by the measure of skin folds at seven sites. Muscle strength/endurance was evaluated by push-up and sit-up tests. Hamstring flexibility was determined using sit-and-reach test. The 12-minutes Cooper test was performed to estimate cardio respiratory fitness of the subjects. Participants that attended at least 75% of the total yoga training sessions were included in the study results. The results of the study showed 1.3 (1.0 - 4.0) cm decrease in WC and 0.7 (0.9 - 1.5) decrease in body fat percentage, and 7.8 (2.0 - 5.0) cm increase in hamstring flexibility and 3.0 (1.0 - 4.0) in abdominal endurance, after the yoga training ($p < 0.01$). In conclusion, the present study results showed that a 12-week yoga program improved physical fitness.

Singh (2017) assessed the effect of yoga on selected physiological variables of female athletes and non athletes. To achieve the objectives of the study one hundred female athletes and one hundred non athletes were randomly selected from the schools of Lucknow Uttar Pradesh as the subjects of the study. All selected subjects were divided randomly into total four groups: two groups female athletes and two groups non athletes (50 each) i.e. one experimental group and one control group for Athlete and one experimental and one control group for non- athlete. The ages of the subjects ranged between 12 to 16 years. Resting heart rate, resting respiratory rate, positive breath holding capacity and negative breath holding capacity were selected as the physiological variables of the study. Resting heart rate recorded as the number of heart beats per minute during the state of proper rest. Resting respiratory rate assessed by rate of respiration in unit counts per minute by carefully watching the moment of the stomach. Positive breath holding capacity recorded as the time of retaining the breath recorded to the nearest second. Negative breath holding capacity recorded as the time of holding the breath recorded to the nearest second. In order to determine the effect of pranadharana on selected physiological variables, analysis of covariance were applied at 0.05 level of significance. The results of the study showed that Pranadharana had no significant effect on the certain Physiological Variables. Pranadharana showed no considerable effect on resting respiratory rate in both experimental groups and control groups. Pranadharana did not significantly affect the resting heart rate. Pranadharana has no significant effect on Positive breath holding capacity. Pranadharana has no significant effect on negative breath holding capacity.

Vishnu (2017) investigated the impact of yogic practices on physical and physiological parameters of college male handball players. To achieve the objectives of the study total 30 inter-collegiate male handball players were selected from affiliated colleges of Bharathiar University, Coimbatore. The subjects were randomly assigned into two equal groups (n=15). Group- I for yogic practices (YPG) and Group- II was worked as a control group (CG). The yoga training program was given to the experimental group for 3 days in a week (Monday, Wednesday and Friday) for the period of 12 weeks. The control group was not assigned to any sort of training except their routine works. A pilot study was conducted to determine the initial capacity of the subjects in order to fix the training load. The physical fitness parameters included shoulder strength (Push-ups) and physiological parameters (Breath Holding Time, Resting Heart Rate) were measured prior and after the training period. The data collected from the subjects was statistically analyzed with „t"test to find out considerable effects if any at 0.05 level of confidence. The result of the shoulder strength, and Breath Holding Time, Resting Heart Rate were significantly improved due to influence of yogic practices with the limitations of (diet, climate, life style) status and previous training. The results of the present study were similar findings of the investigation done by different researchers in the field of sports sciences. Yoga training group significantly improved shoulder strength, and Breath Holding Time, Resting Heart Rate college male handball players.

Kasparavičiūtė et al. (2018) determined the effect of hatha yoga on psychoemotional characteristics of healthy people. Most of the researchers used self-reported methods to evaluate psychoemotional factors. In this study objective method was used to find out what kind of effect could be initiated on psychoemotional characteristics of yoga practitioners. Psychomotoric tone, extra-introversity, aggression, emotional labiality and anxiety were selected as the variables of the study. To achieve the purpose of the study total 40 healthy persons with no reported diseases were selected as the subjects in the research. They were divided into two groups: beginners (practicing yoga for not more than one year, n = 22) and advanced (practicing yoga for at least two years, n = 18) yoga practitioners. Psychoemotional characteristics: innate and present psychomotoric tone, extra-introversity, aggression, emotional lability and anxiety were evaluated using the Myokinetic Psyhodiagnosis of D. Emilio Mira (Simon, 1943) test. The research data was compared with standard limits of score and between the beginners and highly developed yoga practitioners groups. Results of the study showed that Hatha yoga had general effect on psychoemotional status in the beginners and advanced yoga practitioners. Psychomotoric tone improved and emotional lability decreased in both groups significantly ($p < 0.05$). Psychomotoric tone, extra-introversity and emotional lability were within the standard limits. Anxiety and aggression were decreased in both groups in 6-months period. Aggression and emotional lability in the beginners" group was lesser compared to those in the advanced yoga group ($p < 0.05$). Discussion and conclusions of the study: Almost all psychoemotional characteristics were within their standard limits in both groups of yoga practitioners. The higher effect of hatha yoga was originated in the yoga beginners" group.

Shivagumar (2018) assessed the effect of physical exercises and yogic practices on VO2 max and Breath holding time of college level boys. Total 60 college students were selected as the subjects of the study. Their age ranged from 18 to 21 years. Subjects (n=60) were randomly divided into three equal groups of twenty subjects into each group. The experimental group1 assigned to participate in physical exercises and Group 2 yoga group participated in yoga training practices for alternative days per week for a period of six weeks. Group 3 was treated as a control group. All selected subjects of three groups were tested in pre and post of the trainings. Collected Data was statistically examined by analysis of covariance (ANCOVA) and the level of significance was fixed at 0.05 level of confidence to test the F-ratio obtained by analysis of covariance. The results of the study showed that physical exercises group and yoga training group significantly enhanced VO2 max and Breath holding time. So the results support that both physical exercises and yoga are advantageous for physiological variables and health related fitness.

Banerjee et al. (2019) determined the effects of yoga training on physical health and various hematological parameters. To achieve the purpose of the study thirty five healthy individuals (19 Male and 16 Female) selected as the subjects. The age group of subjects were 18 to 45 years participated in the study. They were divided in the study group and the control group. Both groups had same number of subjects in order to minimize the perplexing factors. After a written informed consent, the subjects underwent various types of yoga exercises for 90 days under supervision of qualified yoga trainer. Impact of yoga on body mass index (BMI), pulse rate, blood pressure (BP), and haematological parameters like hemoglobin percentage, white blood cell (WBC) count, platelet count, were taken under consideration prior and after yoga training. Paired t-test was used for statistical analysis. It was observed in the results of the study that BMI, systolic and diastolic BP, and Hb% changed after yoga training significantly. WBC and platelets showed improvement in values after yoga practice but it was statistically non-significant. This study results shows that yoga has beneficial effects on health. The addition of regular yoga exercises with modern medicine in resource-strained public health systems might play a very vital role to provide us a holistic health care.

Mahajan et al. (2019) evaluated the effects of yoga on cardiorespiratory parameters in healthy subjects in South Gujarat region. This study was conducted on age-matched healthy individuals (n = 80) with the age group of 25–60 years. They were divided into control group (n = 40) and yoga group (n = 40). Yoga exercises training was given to yoga group for 10 weeks continuously. Weight, chest girth, chest expansion, pulse rate, blood pressure, RR, tidal volume, breath holding time, vital capacity, expiratory pressure, Population Foundation of India (PFI), and work done were selected as the variables of the study. All selected parameters were measured in both the groups before and after the yogic intervention. Data were compared using Chi-square test. $P < 0.05$ was considered for the statistical significance. Results of the study showed that after 10 weeks of yogic exercise, there was non-significant difference in the mean value of body weight ($P = 0.813$), chest girth ($P = 0.8172$), and chest expansion ($P = 0.7918$). in the same way, the control group also did not show any significant change in these variables. Yoga group showed significant decrease in PR ($P < 0.001$), systolic BP ($P < 0.001$), and diastolic BP ($P < 0.001$). In the control group, the change was insignificant ($P < 0.907$). respiratory rate in the yoga group fell from a mean value of 17.26 ± 2.3 to 13.9 ± 1.4 ($P < 0.001$) while the control group did not show significant changes., fitness index as assessed by Harvard step test showed improvement in the yoga group ($P < 0.05$).

Nandre and Patole (2019) evaluated the effect of suryanamaskara on flexibility, BMI and anaemia in underweight anaemic college level students. For this study, total 50 underweight (BMI < 18.50) and anaemic students age ranged between 18-

22 years were selected randomly as the subjects from Senior College, Pimpalner, Distt. Dhule (MS). They were ready willingly to participate in the study. They were divided into an experimental group and a control group. Yogic trainings were gradually introduced to the experimental group on 6 day in a week for 60 days program from 1st Nov. to 30th Dec.2018. Each training session was nearly 60 to 70 minutes. The treatment was carried out in the evening from 5.30 pm to 6.45 pm. The control group did not performed any yogic exercise. Data collection has been done before and after study for the Variables like flexibility, height, weight and Hb% for both groups. After the Yoga training every subject showed significant positive enhancement in flexibility, weight gaining and Hb level among experimental group when compared to the control group.

Yamamoto et al. (2019) examined the effects of 8 weeks of asana training and asana & Pranayama combination training in order to elucidate the influence of two different combinations of yoga practice on physical and respiratory functions in healthy inactive middle-aged individuals. Total 28 participants (mean age: 52.7 years) were selected for the study. They were divided into the yoga asana (YA) group and asana with pranayama (YAP) group. Participants joined a 70-min session once a week for 8 weeks. The yoga asana group practiced basic asana exercises without specific breathing directives, while the Asana with Pranayama group, combined exercises group practiced basic asana with specific breathing directions (Pranayama). Respiratory function was measured with an auto spirometer. Physical function included the 30-s chair stand test and upper and lower extremity flexibility. All tests were assessed at prior and after 8 weeks of intervention. Changes in variables were analyzed with the paired t-test for both groups. Pre-post results were compared for all the calculated values. $P < 0.05$ was considered statistically considerable. Results of the study showed that both groups have significant improvements in physical and overall respiratory functions after the 8-week yoga trainings. However, the maximal inspiratory pressure and lower extremity flexibility improved significantly only in the Asana with Pranayama group. Conclusions of the study: The 8-week yoga exercises for healthy inactive middle-aged people improved the overall respiratory and physical functions, and the mixture of pranayama had the extra benefits of improving inspiratory muscle strength and overall body flexibility.

Bhowmik and Kumar (2020) evaluated the outcome of yoga training on resting heart rate (RHR), peak expiratory flow rate (PEFR) and body mass index (BMI) among rural school boys of West Bengal and Western Uttar Pradesh (W.U.P.). Total twenty (20) rural school boys (height 1.45 ± 0.06 mts and weight 41.42 ± 7.47 kg) of West Bengal state and 20 rural school boys (height 1.46 ± 0.05 mts. and weight 42.32 ± 6.76 kg) of Western Uttar Pradesh state were randomly selected as subjects of the study. All subjects were students of the class 6th to 8th. Subjects of both places participated in yoga training for 16 weeks period. The resting heart rate, peak expiratory flow rate and body mass index (BMI) were measured before and after training treatment. The data was analyzed by using t-test and significant level was set at $p < 0.05$. Results of the study showed that after the yoga training resting heart rate significantly reduced, Peak expiratory flow rate significantly improved and BMI no changed between the school boys of W.B and W.U.P. Conclusion: the same yoga training significantly reduced resting heart rate and improved peak expiatory flow rate between class 6th to 8th standard students of different civilizing and geographical areas in India.

SUMMARY OF THE LITERATURE REVIEW:

The researcher collected as many as possible reviews related to the effects of yoga exercises. The literature analysed consisted of different approaches and concentrating on the effect of yoga/ hatha yoga trainings on physical fitness, physiological and biochemical or haematological variables. These studies were collected from Panjab University Chandigarh, M.D.U. Rohtak libraries and on the internet from Research gate, Shodhganga INFLEBNET, Taylor and Francis, Medline/PubMed, google scholar, Scopus journals, and other online sources to give sufficient knowledge to the readers and for the effective analysis of the present study. The literature available so far is not conclusive to consider the effect of Hatha yoga on physical fitness, physiological and haematological variables of school level students. The review of related literature has helped the researcher to formulate the present problem. On the bases of knowledge gained from the review of literature and dialogue with relevant experts, the researcher framed an appropriate methodology to be applied to research, which is presented in chapter III.

CHAPTER-III

METHOD AND PROCEDURE

In this chapter the Methodology used for the study has been explained. Design of the study selection of subjects, selection of variables, Selection of tests, Criterion measures, reliability of data, instrumental reliability, tester`s reliability, pilot study, training programmes, administration of tests, collection of data and statistical procedure that were used have been presented here.

DESIGN OF THE STUDY: The present study was an experimental type of study to find out the effect of hatha yoga on physical fitness, physiological, and haematological variables of school level students.

Figure 3.1 Flow chart showing the methodology adopted in this study.

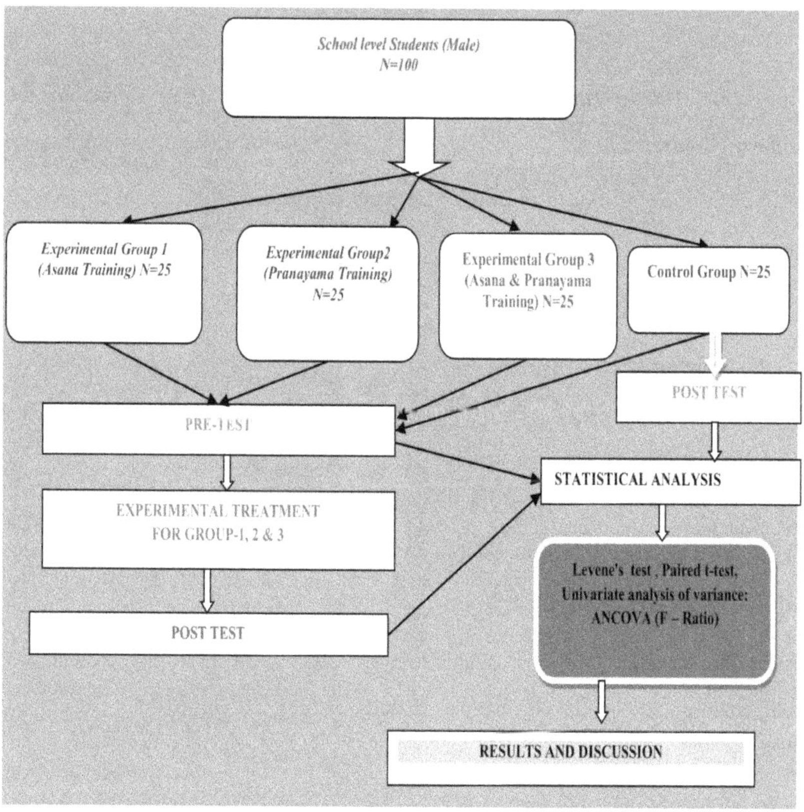

SELECTION OF SUBJECTS:

With the help of purposive sampling (Non-probability sampling) total 100 male students out of total 265 students of 9th to 12th classes, from Govt. Sr. Sec. School Ugalan, District Hisar (Haryana) were selected as the subjects to achieve the purpose of this study. They were divided into four equal groups randomly with consisting of 25 subjects in each group. Experiment Group I underwent yoga asana training (AT), Group II was subjected to pranayamas training (PT) and group III was given yoga asana and pranayamas combination training for the duration of 12 weeks with five days per week while group IV was monitored as control group. The control group did not participate in any training program. A qualified physician examined the basic health of the selected subjects and declared them fit for the study. All subjects were informed about the purpose and nature of the study in detail. Consent was obtained by the parents of the subjects because maximum numbers of students were under the age of 18 years.

Figure 3.2 The detailed distribution of the sample has been shown in the following figure:

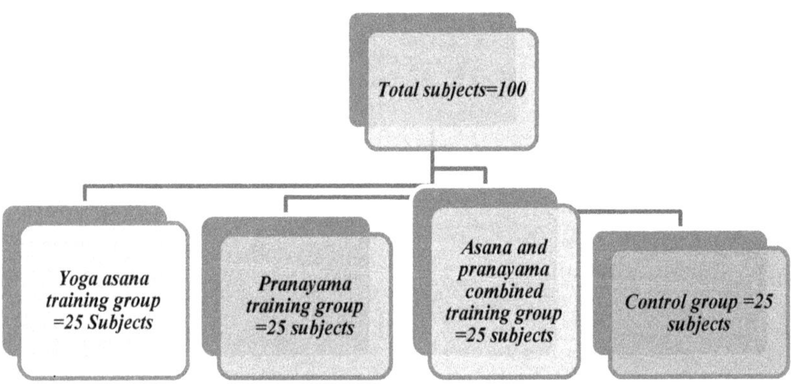

SELECTION OF VARIABLES:

Under the guidance and in Consultation with experts the following criteria was considered in selecting the variables of the study.

- Tester`s capability.
- Feasibility criteria in mind.

- ❖ Especially equipment"s reliability and time factor.
- ❖ Basis of available literature.
- ❖ Keeping the specific purpose of the study.

DEPENDENT VARIABLES:

The following physical fitness, physiological and haematological variables were selected for the experiment for analysis.

PHYSICAL FITNESS VARIABLES (Components):

1. Speed
2. Strength
3. Agility
4. Flexibility
5. Endurance

PHYSIOLOGICAL VARIABLES (Components):

1. Systolic blood pressure
2. Diastolic blood pressure
3. Resting heart rate
4. Breath holding capacity

HAEMATOLOGICAL VARIABLES (Components):

1. White blood cell
2. Red blood cell
3. Haemoglobin
4. Platelets count

INDEPENDENT VARIABLES:

The following Hatha Yoga Trainings were considered as the independent variables.

1. Asana Training (AT).
2. Pranayama Training (PT).
3. Asana & Pranayama combined Training (APT).

SELECTION OF TESTS:

The purpose of this study was to assess the effect of hatha yoga on physical, physiological and haematological variables. The following test was selected to measure the variables

PHYSICAL FITNESS TESTS:

To test the physical fitness of the students AAHPHER YOUTH FITNESS TEST BATTERY (1976) was used and to test the flexibility AAHPERD (1980) test was used for following physical fitness variables.

1. Speed – 50 Mts. dash running
2. Strength – Standing broad jump
3. Agility – shuttle run
4. Flexibility – Sit and Reach
5. Endurance - 12 Minutes walk /run

PHYSIOLOGICAL VARIABLES TESTS:

1. Systolic blood pressure – Sphygmomanometer, Stethoscope
2. Diastolic blood pressure - Sphygmomanometer, Stethoscope
3. Resting heart rate – Stop watch
4. Breath holding time – Stop watch

HAEMATOLOGICAL VARIABLES TEST:

1. White blood cell
2. Red blood cell
3. Haemoglobin
4. Platelets count

(White blood cell, Red blood cell, Haemoglobin: Complete Blood Count (CBC) Test.)

All haematological variables were measured in a medical Laboratory by CBC Test.

CRITERION MEASURES:

The following criterion measures were used for testing the hypothesis:

Table 3.1 Selected variables, unit, test and equipments.

	Selected Variables	**Unit**	*Test and Equipment*
Physical fitness Variables	Speed	Second	50 Mts. Dash Run
	Strength	Meter	Standing broad jump
	Agility	Second	Shuttle Run
	Flexibility	Centimeters	Sit and Reach
	Endurance	Meter	Cooper test run/walk (12 Minutes)
Physiological Variables	Systolic blood pressure	MmHg	Stethoscope and Sphygmomanometer
	Diastolic blood pressure	MmHg	Stethoscope & Sphygmomanometer
	Resting heart rate	Beats/minute	Stop watch
	Breath Holding time	Seconds	Stop watch
Haematological variable	White blood cell	10^3/uL	Blood sample (CBC Test)
	Red blood cell	10^6/uL	Blood sample (CBC Test)
	Hemoglobin	g/Dl	Blood sample (CBC Test)
	Platelets count	10^3/uL	Blood sample (CBC Test)

ORIENTATION OF THE SUBJECTS:

Prior to pre- test and trainings the researcher explained to the subjects about the purpose of the study. The researcher also explained very deeply about Asana training, Pranayama training and combined training of Asana & Pranayama. He explained the benefits of the trainings to the subjects. The method and value of each yoga exercises which were included in the trainings were performed and explained first by investigator. The researcher motivated the subjects for full co-operation and involve completely in their respective training to achieve maximum output.

INSTRUMENTAL RELIABLITY:

The instruments which were used and operated for this study to examine the variables were aligned and institutionalized or standardized. These tools were taken from the department of Physical Education, Panjab University, Chandigarh and other different establishments.

TESTER`S COMPETENCY AND RELIABILITY OF TEST:

To ensure the tester`s competency the tester had a number of practice sessions and made testing strategy. Every test item was conducted by the tester when subjects were very much conversant with tests and their methodology.

RELIABILITY OF THE DATA:

To validate the scoring techniques were used in the research work for different physical fitness parameters, physiological parameters of students test –retest method of reliability was administered on 10 students.

Table 3.2 Reliability co-efficient of physical fitness variable.

(n-10)

Sr.no.	Physical fitness Parameter	Co-efficient of reliability
1.	Speed (sec.)	0.979
2.	Strength (m.)	0.923
3.	Agility (Sec.)	0.965
4.	Flexibility	0.989
5.	Endurance (m)	0.937

*Significant at 0.05 level

The table 3.2 showed the reliability of physical fitness variables. Reliability of speed was 97.9%, reliability of strength was 92.3%, reliability of agility was 96.5%, reliability of flexibility was 98.9% and reliability of endurance was 93.7%,

Table 3.3 Reliability co-efficient of physiological parameters

(n-10)

Sr.no.	Physiological Parameter	Co-efficient of reliability
1.	Systolic blood pressure	0.947
2.	Diastolic blood pressure	0.955
3.	Resting heart rate	0.998
4.	Breath holding time	0.969

*Significant at 0.05 level

Table 3.3 shows reliability co-efficient of selected physiological parameters used in the study. Least reliability was observed as 94.7% for systolic blood pressure. All physiological variables had good reliability co-efficient.

PILOT STUDY

A pilot study was conducted on total 15 students before finalizing the training program to ensure that the intensity and duration of the activities included in the five subjects for yoga asana, five subjects for pranayamas and five subjects for combination of asana and pranayamas training program were within the limits of the subjects capacity to produce the desired effects.

TRAINING PROGRAMME

To achieve the objectives of the study the experimental groups underwent their respective training programmes.

- **Experimental Group I : Underwent Asana Training (AT).**
- **Experimental Group II : Underwent Pranayama Training (PT)**
- **Experimental Group III : Underwent Asana & Pranayama Training (APT).**
- **Control Group IV : No Specific Training Programme**

The training programs were scheduled with the duration and load which was based on the result of the pilot study. The training programs were carried out for a period of 12 weeks. Training was given for five day per week. Control group did not take part in any specific training programme apart from their daily routine. All subjects were instructed by researcher not to change their life and dietary habits for the entire period of training. Every training session was 50 minutes. The training program was scheduled in the morning between 6.00am to 7.00am from Monday to Friday. The subjects were participated their respective program under strict supervision of researcher. Three yoga experts assisted the researcher during training session. One expert helped yoga asana training group, the second expert assigned for pranayamas training group, and the third expert helped combined group of asana and pranayamas training. All three yoga assistants strictly followed their training programs respectively. Subjects would undergoing a 10 minutes warming up exercises, which was included on the spot jogging, inhale and exhale breath as possible as long, neck rotations, arms stretching, shoulder rotation, spine stretching exercises, push-ups etc. and 10 minutes cooling down exercises which included supine spinal twists, neck rotations, arms stretching, savasana and easy pose etc.

ASANA GROUP TRAINING PRORAM

Asana training group underwent asana training for five days in a week for twelve weeks. Figure 3.3 flow chart of asana training group and table 3.4 shows detailed programme of asana training.

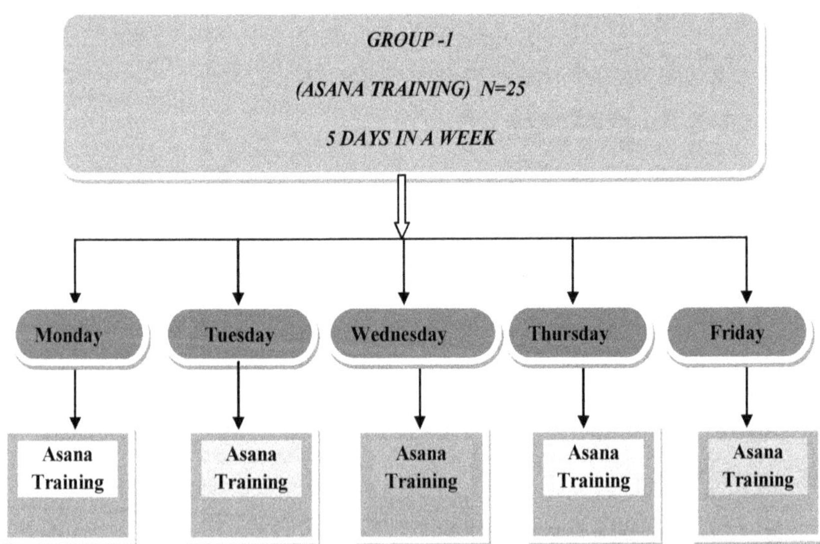

Figure 3.3 Flow chart showing the experimental treatment adopted for experimental group –I.

Table 3.4 Yoga asana training detailed program.

S.No.	*Name of yoga*	*1 to 4 week*		*5 to 8 week*		*9 to 12 week*	
		Duration	***Rest***	***Duration***	***Rest***	***Duration***	***Rest***
1	Warm up	10 minutes					
2	Tadasana	30 Sec	1Minute.	45Sec.	45 Sec	1Minute	30 Sec.
3	Trikonasana	30 Sec	1Minute	45Sec.	45Sec.	1Minute	30 Sec.
4	Padmasana	30 Sec	1Minute	45Sec.	45Sec.	1Minute	30 Sec.
5	Vajrasana	30 Sec	1Minute	45Sec.	45Sec.	1Minute	30 Sec.
6	Bhujangasana	30 Sec	1Minute	45Sec.	45Sec.	1Minute	30 Sec.
7	Shalabasana	30 Sec	1Minute	45Sec.	45Sec.	1Minute	30 Sec.
8	Dhanurasana	30 Sec	1Minute	45Sec.	45Sec.	1Minute	30 Sec.
9	Halasana	30 Sec	1Minute	45Sec.	45Sec.	1Minute	30 Sec.
10	Chakrasana	30 Sec	1Minute	45Sec.	45Sec.	1Minute	30 Sec.
11	Matsayasana	30 Sec	1Minute	45Sec.	45Sec.	1Minute	30 Sec.
12	Cooling down	10 minutes					

Each training session of yoga asana group had 10 asanas and each asana had 2 repetitions. Training was divided in three phases. Each phase had 4 weeks. In first phase of asana training no holding position took place. Second phase had 15 seconds holding position and in the third phase of training 30 seconds of final position holding took place.

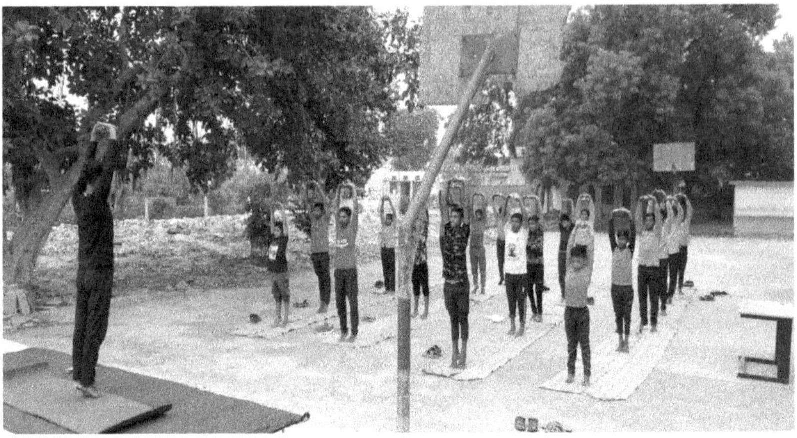

Figure 3.4 Tadasana performed by Asana group

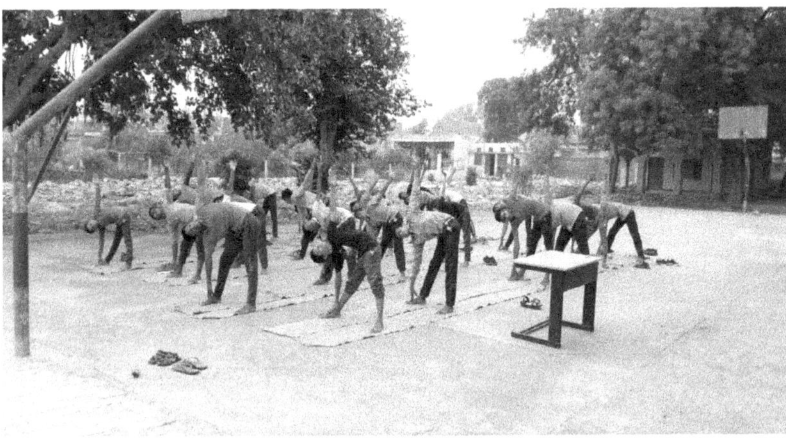

Figure 3.5 Trikonasana performed by Asana group

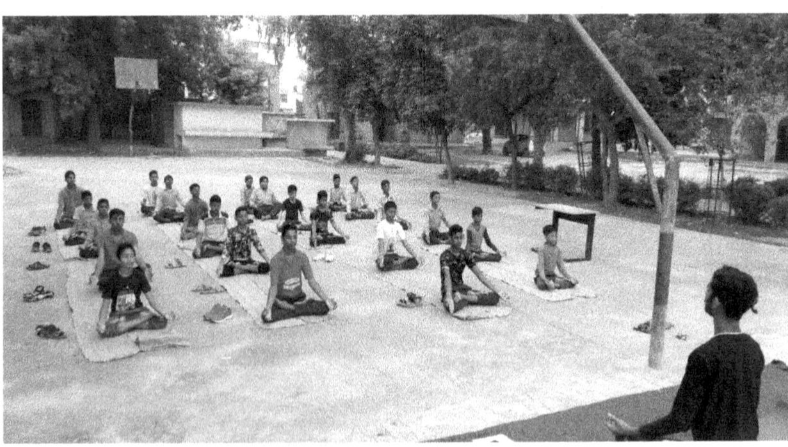

Figure 3.6 Padmasana performed by Asana group

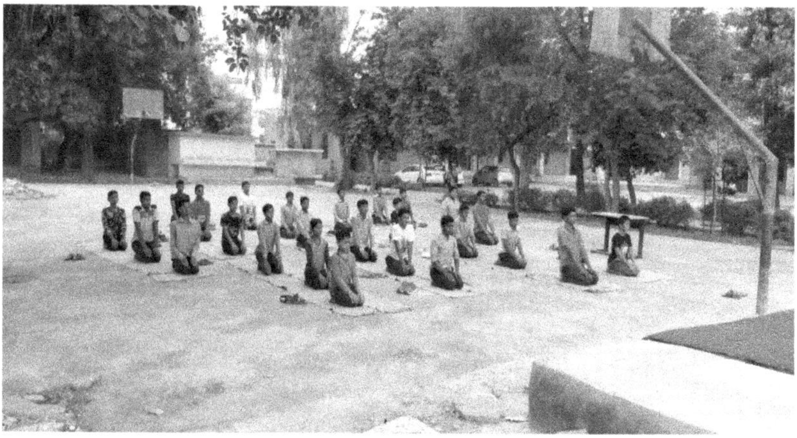

Figure 3.7 Vajrasana performed by Asana group

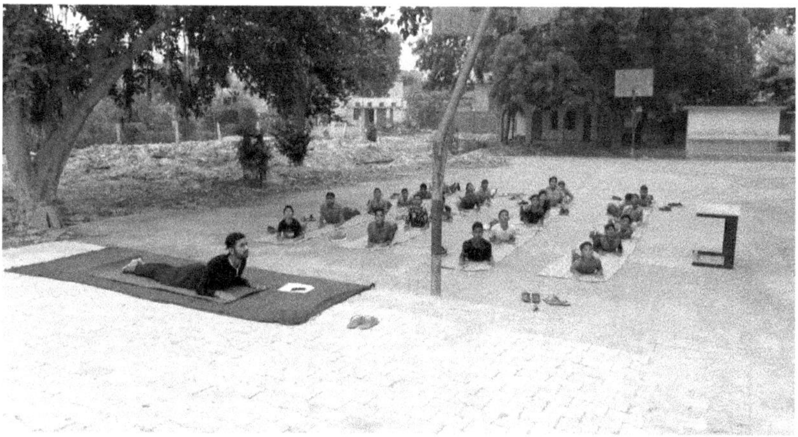

Figure 3.8 Bhujangasana performed by Asana group

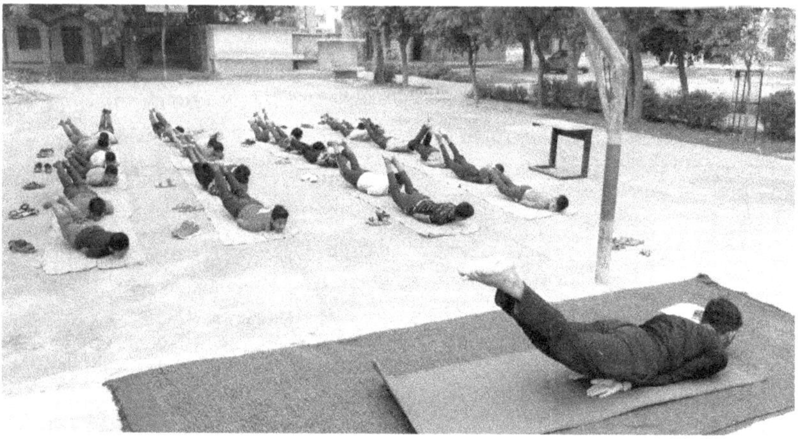

Figure 3.9 Salabhasana performed by Asana group

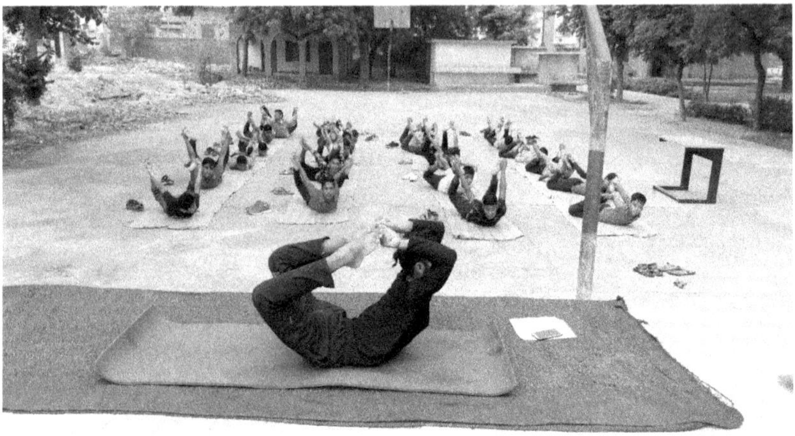

Figure 3.10 Dhanurasana performed by Asana group

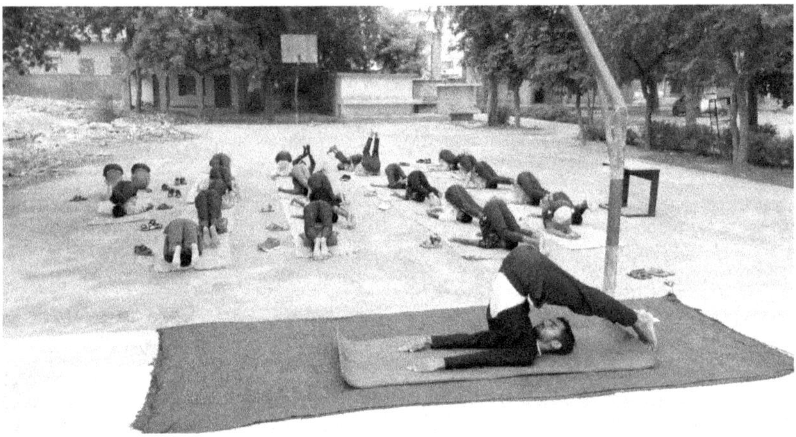

Figure 3.11 Halasana performed by Asana group

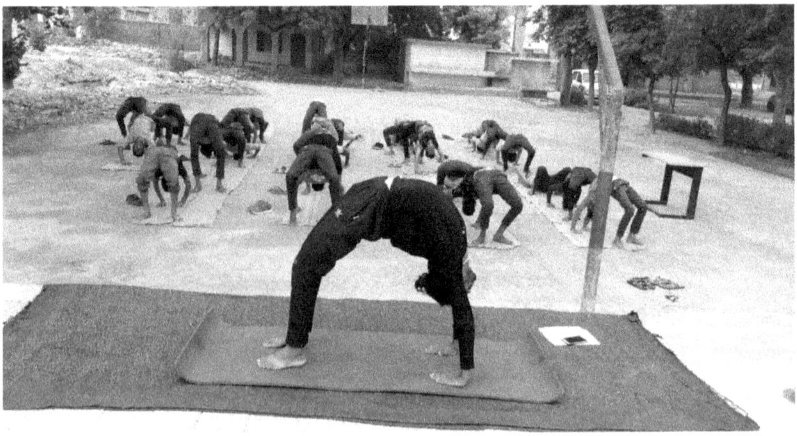

Figure 3.12 Chakrasana performed by Asana group

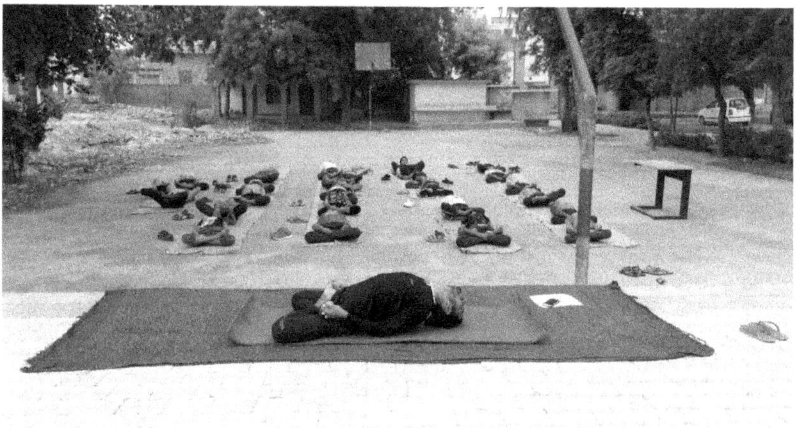

Figure 3.13 Matsayasana performed by Asana Group

PRANAYAMA GROUP TRAINING PROGRAM

Pranayama training group underwent Pranayama training for five days in a week for twelve weeks. Figure 3.14 flow chart of Pranayama training group and table 3.5 shows detailed programme of Pranayama training.

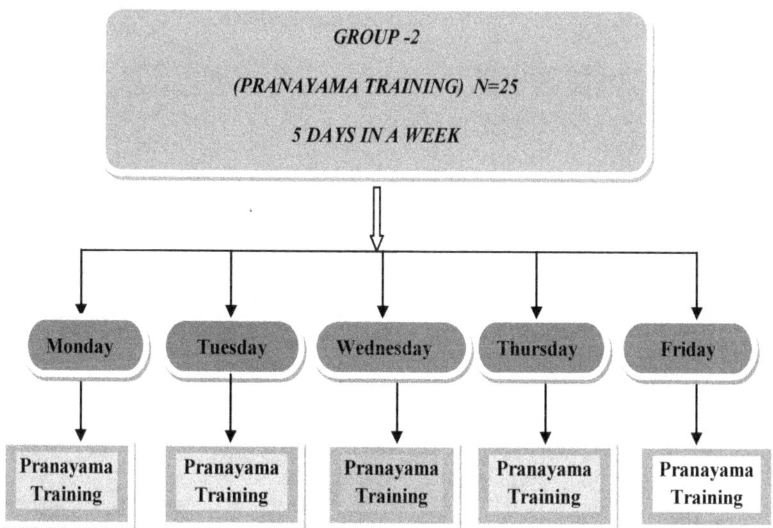

Figure 3.14 Flow chart showing the experimental treatment adopted for experimental group –II.

Table 3.5 Pranayama group training program

S.No.	*Name of pranayama*	*1 to 4 week*		*5 to 8 week*		*9 to 12 week*	
		Duration	***Rest***	***Duration***	***Rest***	***Duration***	***Rest***
1	Warm up	10 minutes					
2	Bhastrika	2 MIN.	3 MIN.	3 MIN	2 MIN.	4 MIN.	1 MIN.
3	Kapalbhati	2 MIN.	3 MIN.	3 MIN	2 MIN.	4 MIN.	1 MIN.
4	Anulom Vilom	2 MIN.	3 MIN.	3 MIN	2 MIN.	4 MIN.	1 MIN.
5	Shitali	2 MIN.	3MIN.	3 MIN	2 MIN.	4 MIN.	1 MIN.
6	Bhramari	2 MIN.	3 MIN	3 MIN	2 MIN.	4 MIN.	1 MIN.
7	Udgeeth	2 MIN.	3 MIN	3 MIN	2 MIN.	4 MIN.	1 MIN.
8	Cooling Down	10 Minutes					

Each training session of pranayamas group had six pranayamas. Training was divided in three phases. Each phase had 4 weeks. In first phase of training duration of each pranayama was 2 minutes and duration of rest was 3 minutes. In second phase duration of pranayama was 3 minutes and rest was 2 minutes and in third phase duration of pranayama was 4 minutes and rest was 1 minute.

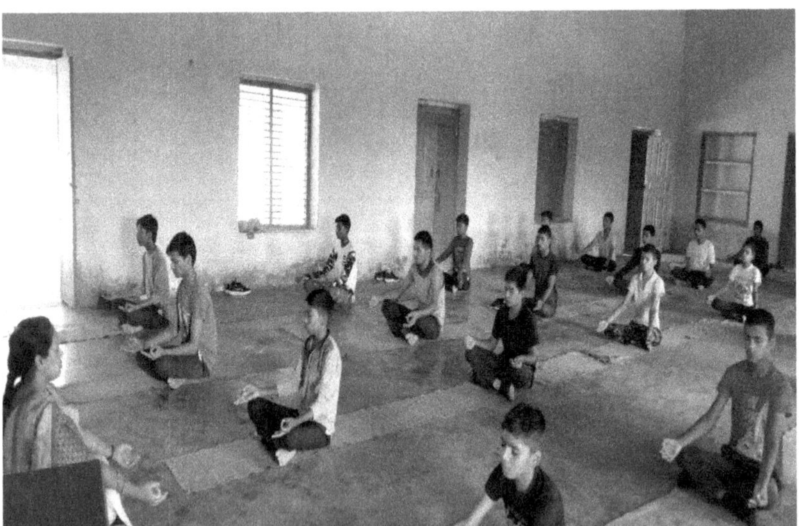

Figure 3.15 Bhastrika performed by Pranayama group

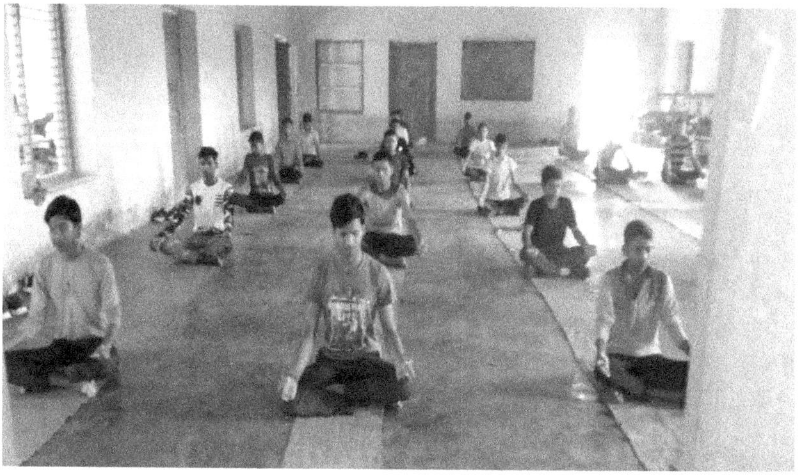

Figure 3.16 Kapalbhati performed by Pranayama group

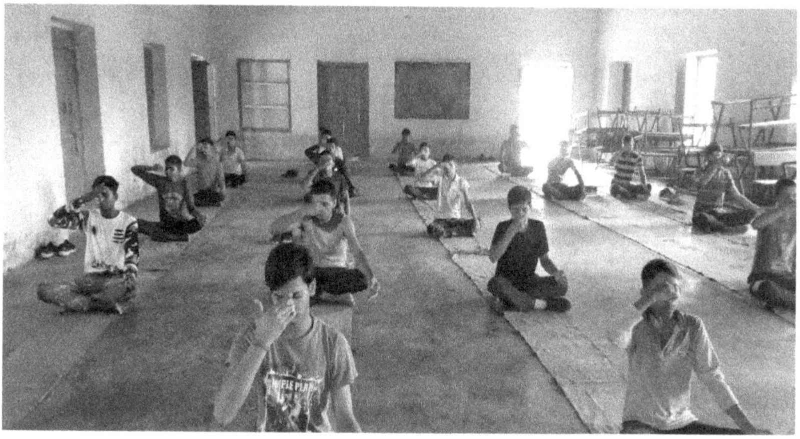

Figure 3.17 Anulom Vilom performed by Pranayama group

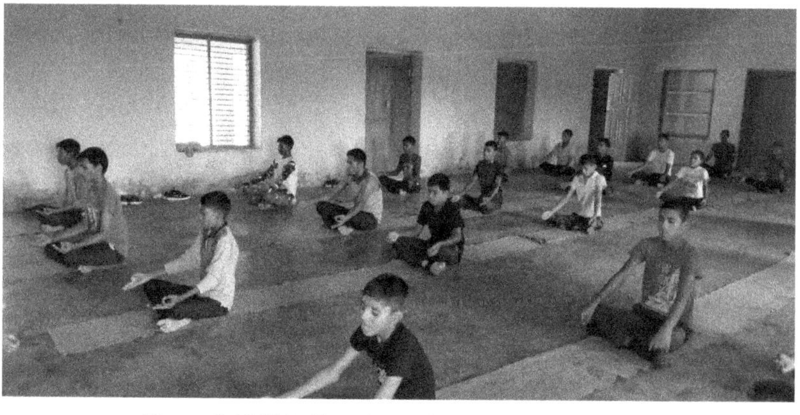

Figure 3.18 Shitali performed by Pranayama group

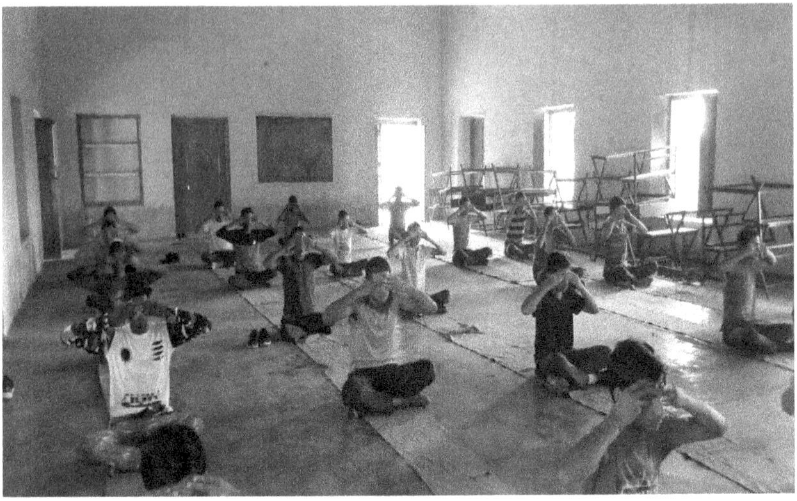

Figure 3.19 Bhramari performed by Pranayama group

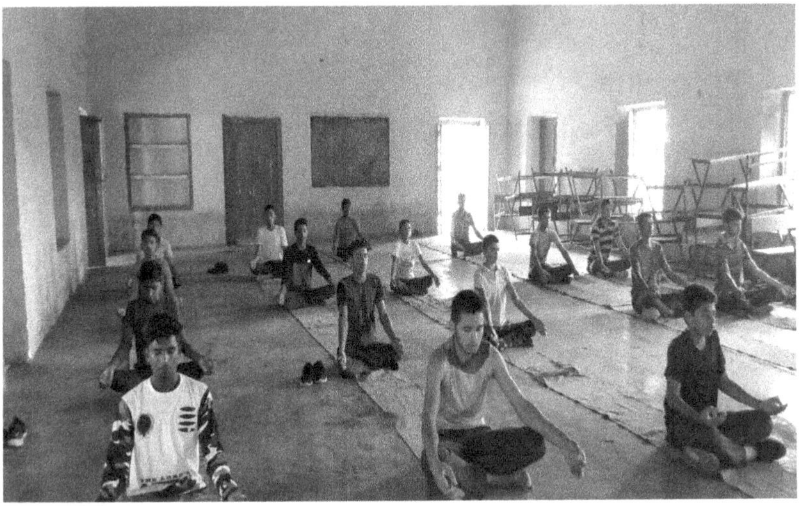

Figure 3.20 Udgeeth performed by Pranayama group

ASANA AND PRANAYAMA COMBINED GROUP TRAINING PROGRAM

Asana & Pranayama training group underwent Asana & Pranayama combined training for five days in a week for twelve weeks. Figure 3.21 flow chart of Asana & Pranayama training group and table 3.6 shows detailed programme of Pranayama training.

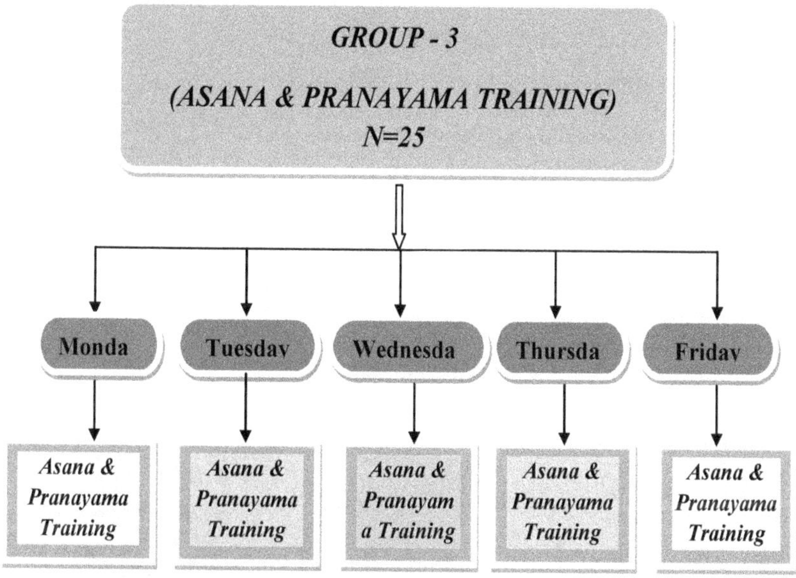

Figure 3.21 Flow chart showing the experimental treatment adopted for experimental group –III

Table 3.6 Asana and pranayama combined group training program.

S.No.	*Name of yoga*	*1 to 4 week*		*5 to 8 week*		*9 to 12 week*	
		Duration	*Rest*	*Duration*	*Rest*	*Duration*	*Rest*
1	Warm up	10 minutes					
2	Tadasana	30 Sec	1Minute	45Sec.	45 Sec	1Minute	30 Sec.
3	Padmasana	30 Sec	1Minute	45Sec.	45Sec.	1Minute	30 Sec.
4	Bhujangasana	30 Sec	1Minute	45Sec.	45Sec.	1Minute	30 Sec.
5	Shalabasana	30 Sec	1Minute	45Sec.	45Sec.	1Minute	30 Sec.
6	Halasana	30 Sec	1Minute	45Sec.	45Sec.	1Minute	30 Sec.
7	Bhastrika	2 MIN.	3 MIN.	3 MIN	2 MIN.	4 MIN.	1 MIN.
8	Anulom Vilom	2 MIN.	3 MIN.	3 MIN	2 MIN.	4 MIN.	1 MIN.
9	Udgeeth	2 MIN.	3 MIN	3 MIN	2 MIN.	4 MIN.	1 MIN.
10	Cooling down	10 minutes					

Each training session of asana and pranayamas combined group had 6 asanas and 3 pranayamas. Training was divided in three phases. Each phase had 4 weeks. Each asana had 2 repetitions and in the first phase no holding position took place. Second phase had 15 seconds holding position and in third phase of training 30 seconds of final position holding took place. In first phase of training duration of each pranayama was 2 minutes and rest was 3 minutes. In second phase duration of pranayama was 3 minutes and rest was 2 minutes and in third phase duration of pranayama was 4 minutes and rest was 1 minute.

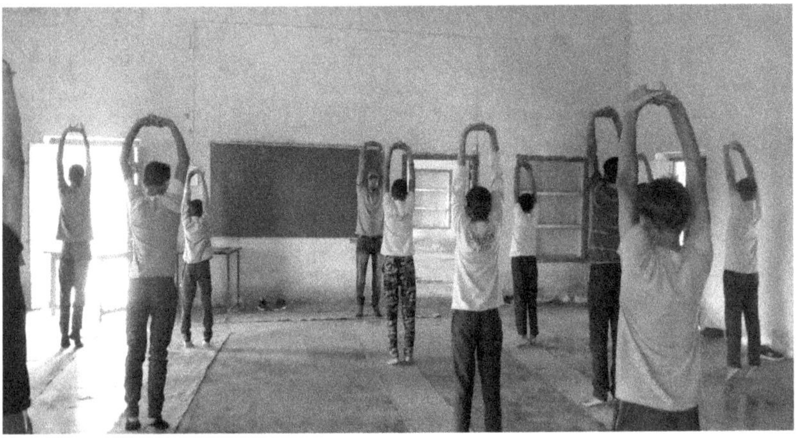

Figure 3.22 Tad asana performed by asana and pranayama combined group

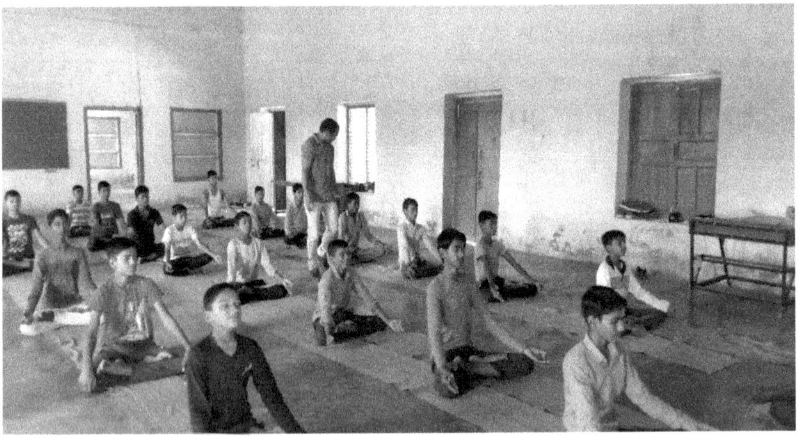

Figure 3.23 Padmasana performed by asana and pranayama combined group

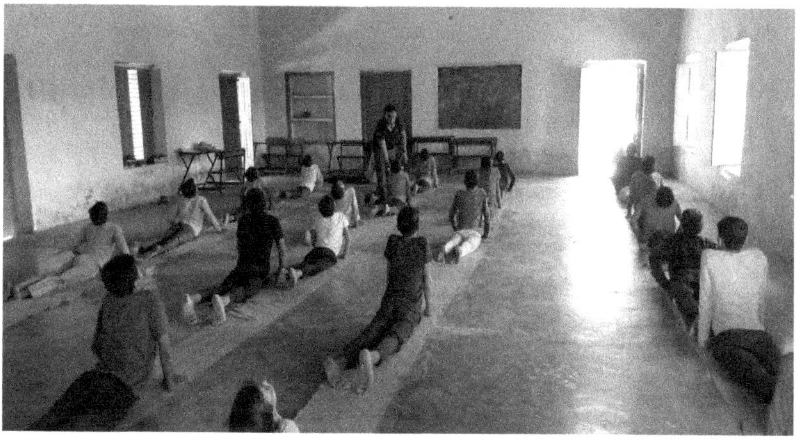

Figure 3.24 Bhujangasana performed by asana and pranayama combined group

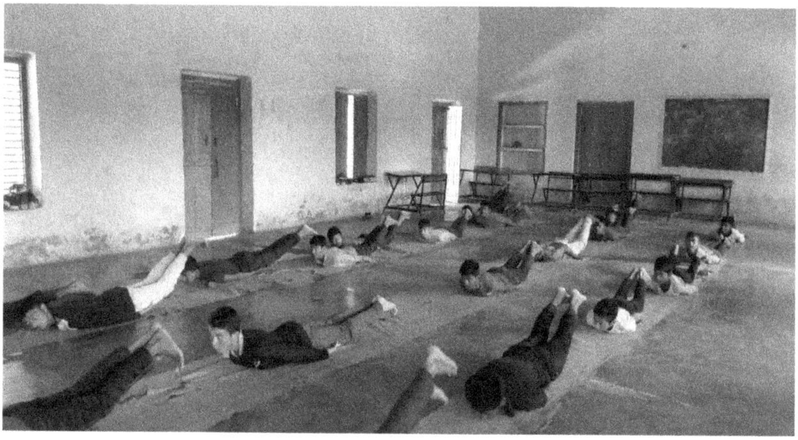

Figure 3.25 Salabhasana performed by asana and pranayama combined group

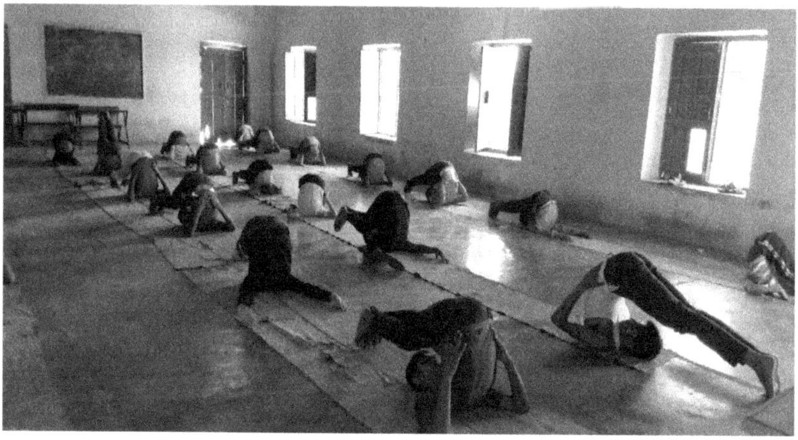

Figure 3.26 Halasana performed by asana and pranayama combined group

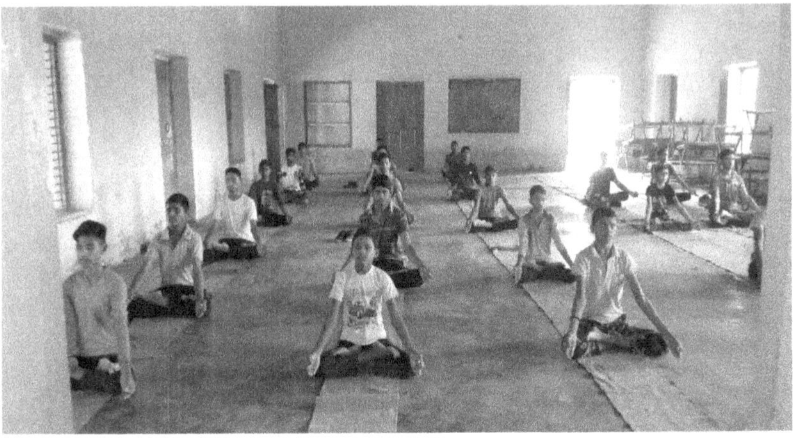

Figure 3.27 Bhastrika performed by asana and pranayama combined group

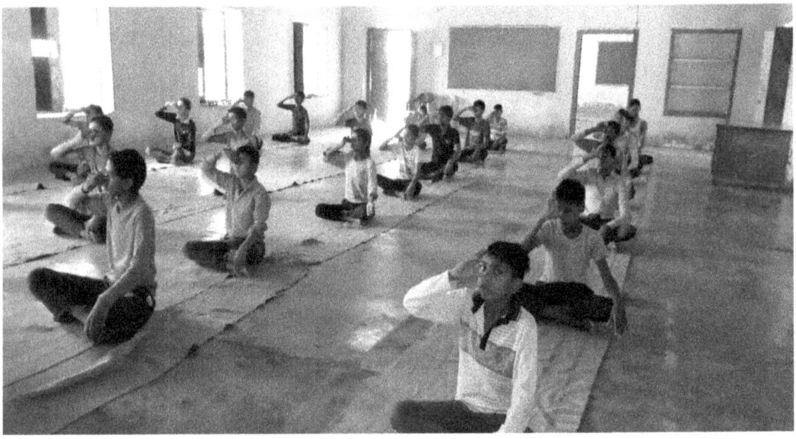

Figure 3.28 AnulomVilom performed by asana and pranayama combined group

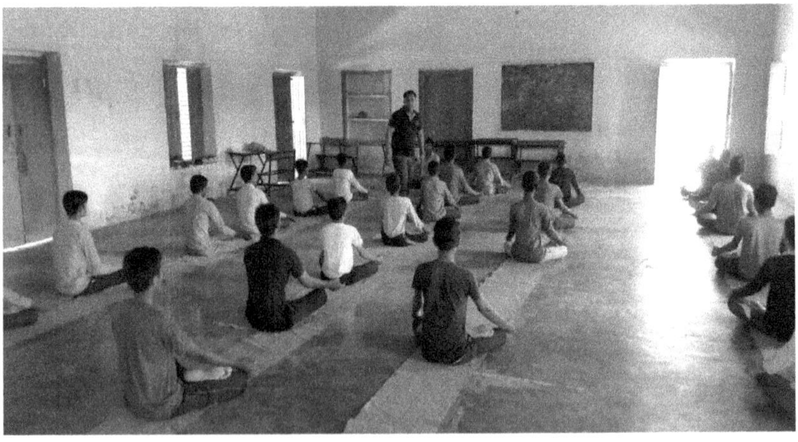

Figure 3.29 Udgeeth performed by asana and pranayama combined group.

HATHA YOGA PRACTICES AND PROCEDURES (USED IN THE STUDY):

ASANA

Tadasana:

In Sanskrit Tada means Mountain so it`s also called Mountain pose. It is very effective for stretching whole body muscles.

Tadasana steps:

- Stand straight. Keeping your back, legs and neck straight.
- Your arms should be hanging alongside with body.
- Start deep inhaling and raise both arms upward.
- Your fingers are interlocked with each other.
- Now raise heels and stand on toes.
- Body in full stretch, feel the stretch from feet to fingers of your arms.
- Hold this position according to your training phase.
- Exhale your breath and come to the initial position.

Trikonasana:

Trikonasana is also known as Triangle pose. It is helpful in maintaining balance and stretch of several muscles in the body.

Trikonasana steps:

- Stand straight and keep distance of approximately 3 feet between your legs.
- Extend your arms sideways with the level of your shoulders.
- Start inhaling, raise the left arm and bend your body towards right.
- Right hand fingers pointing towards your toes.
- Your eyes should be open and face the ceiling.
- Hold your position according to training programme.
- Exhale your breath slowly and come to starting position.
- Repeat the asana for other side.

Padmasana:

Padmasana is also known as "Lotus pose". It is best asana for meditation. Padmasana is a exercise for abdominal and pelvic region. It helps redirect your downward energy.

Padmasana steps:

- Sit on mat with straight legs in front, keeping the spine erect.
- Bend your right knee with holding of both hands and place it on the left thigh.
- Same step repeat with left leg.
- Both of your legs crossed and placed on opposite thighs.
- Place your hands on your knees in mudra position.
- Your face and spine erect. Hold the position with gentle deep breathing.

Vajrasana:

This asana also known as Thunderbolt pose. It is very helpful for our digestive system. It is very beneficial for our back and chest muscles.

Vajrasana steps:

- Sit on your knees with keeping the head and back erect.
- Your toes cross each other.
- Your buttocks placed on the heels and thighs on the calf muscles.
- Your hands on the knees and face focus on straight.
- Keep your attention to the breathing.
- Close your eyes and concentrate on breathing process.
- Hold your position.

Bhujangasana:

Bhujangasana is also known as Cobra pose. It is very beneficial to increase the flexibility of the spine. It strengthens our back muscle and is helpful in relieving back pain. It reduces belly fat and tones up our abdomen.

Bhujangasana steps:

- Lie down on stomach.
- Raise the trunk and head with the support of your palm.
- Bend your elbows and make arch with your neck.
- Look upward and keep your stomach on the floor.
- Put pressure on toes and extend them like a cobra.
- Hold your final position for some time.

Shalabhasana:

Shalbhasana is also known as locust pose. It is helpful in increasing blood circulation in the whole body. It makes us fit and healthy. It reduces the stiffness of the back.

Shalabhasana steps:

- Lie down on the ground on stomach and put your palms on the ground.
- Make sure your both feet join each other.
- Inhale the breath slowly and raise your lower portion of the waist and keep the legs straight.
- Your both hands are put on the beneath of the stomach.
- Hold this position for some time.

Dhanurasana:

Dhanurasana gets this name from Sanskrit words "Dhanu" which means a Bow. In this asana your body looks like a bow. Regular exercise of this asana stretches all the muscles of the body. It also strengthens our back muscles and improves flexibility.

Dhanurasana steps:

- Lie down on the ground on your stomach and your arms placed beside the body.
- Your feet apart with hip width.
- Fold your knees and try to place ankles on buttocks.
- Hold your ankles and try to lift chest and thighs.

- Hold this position.
- To get out of the posture, leave your ankle and lay down again.

Halasana:

This name comes from Sanskrit two words "Hal" means Plow and asana means posture. Plow is a farming tool. It makes the spine strong and flexible. It also strengthens the neck muscles.

Halasana steps:

- Lie on the back, your legs close together and arms placed beside the body.
- Place your palms on the floor.
- Take deep breath and raise your both legs up.
- Raise your buttock and touch the floor with the toes.
- Hold your position.
- Raise the legs and lowering the back roll over to your initial position.

Chakrasana:

Chakrasana known as wheel pose. This name is derived from Sanskrit word chakra which means wheel. It is backward bending asana which increases the flexibility of the spine.

Chkrasana steps:

- Lie down on the yoga mat and place your feet apart.
- Bend your knees and place on the ground close to your buttocks.
- Your palm just under the shoulders and elbows placed with the shoulder width.
- Take deep breath and put pressure on palms as they touch the floor.
- Lift your elbows and shoulders from the ground.
- Slowly lift your hips up and roll your spine like a semi circle arch.
- Stay in this position.
- In order to come to initial position bend the elbows and lower your shoulders.
- Bring the hips and spine back to the surface of ground.

Matsayasana:

In this asana your body takes the shape like a fish. This asana is known as the destroyer of all diseases. It stretches our spine and muscles. It helps to attain the body mind balance.

Matsayasana steps:

- Sit in padmasana and take deep breath.
- Bend backward without releasing padmasana posture.
- Take support of your elbows and try to touch your head to the floor.
- Try to arch your spine and hold your toes with hands.
- Keep your eyes open and hold this position.
- Slowly come back in initial position.

PRANAYAMA:

Bhastrika Pranayama:

Bhastrika Pranayama is an important breath exercise in yoga. It involves a deep and forceful process of inhalation and exhalation of breath. It helps in balancing Vata, Pitta and Kapha.

Bhastrika Steps:

- Sit in Padmasana.
- Keep your spine and neck erect.
- Take a long and deep breath.
- Fill your lungs with air and hold breath sometime.
- Exhale the breath and repeat the process.

Kapalbhati Pranayama:

Kapalbhati name comes from Sanskrit words Kapal and bhati. Kapal means forehead and Bhati means shining. So it is also called skull shining breathing technique. It is helpful in releasing all toxins of our body.

Kapalbhati steps:

- Sit comfortably in padmasana
- Take a deep long breath in.
- Pull your stomach when you exhale.
- Do it as much as you comfortably can.
- In inhalation the breath flows into lungs automatically.
- Repeat this process again and again.

Anulom Vilom Pranayama:

It is an alternate breathing exercise. It is very beneficial for our respiratory and cardiovascular system. Regular practice of anulom vilom improves lung function and endurance.

Anulom Vilom Steps:

- Sit in a meditation pose and keep your spine straight.
- Close your eyes and using your right hand, fold middle and index fingers toward palm.
- Place your thumb on your right nostril and close it.
- Inhale through your left nostril deeply and hold it.
- Release your thumb and close your left nostril with ring finger.
- Exhale through the right nostril.
- Now in reverse process inhaling through the right nostril and exhaling through the left nostril.

Shitali Pranayama:

Shitali Pranayama cools our body and also helps in relaxing the nerves and muscles. It is also beneficial for high blood pressure patients.

Shitali Pranayama Steps:

- Sit in any comfortable pose.
- Keep your back and neck erect.

- Close your eyes and roll up your tongue and make its shape like a tube.
- Inhale maximum air through your tongue.
- Close your mouth and exhale through your nose.
- Repeat all this process again and again.

Bhramari Pranayama:

The name Bhramari derives from the Indian black bee called "Bhramar". It is one of the best pranayama exercises to free the mind of agitation and frustration. In this pranayama a typical humming sound of a bee is produced when we exhale.

Bhramari steps:

- Sit up with straight back and neck on the ground.
- Close your eyes and keep the mind calm.
- Plug both the ears with using the thumbs and the eyes are kept closed by middle fingers.
- Start deep inhaling through nose and hold breath for some seconds.
- Start creating sound from the throat when exhale and the sound similar to the humming sound of the bee.

Udgeeth Pranayama:

It is most easy and common breathing exercise among all Pranayama exercises. It is the art of conscious breathing. This Pranayama involves chanting of sound "OM" with every exhalation.

Udgeeth Pranayama steps:

- Sit on the padmasana with straight spine.
- Close your eyes.
- Inhale deeply through your nostrils till your lungs are full with air.
- While exhaling chants the word Om, keep the sound „O" long and „M" short.
- Repeat the process according to your training programme.

ADMINISTRATION OF TESTS:

PHYSICAL FITNESS VARIABLES

SPEED (50m DASH)

Objective: To measure the speed of the subjects.

Facilities and Equipments required: Track, measuring tape, whistle/clapper and stop watch. (Calibrated to 1/100 seconds)

Procedure and scoring: The subjects were requested to stand behind the starting line and given instructions to start with a standing start position. On hearing the whistle/clapper sound, the subject had to run with his maximum speed and effort to cross the finishing line as soon as possible. The best time out of two trials was recorded as the subject individual"s score.

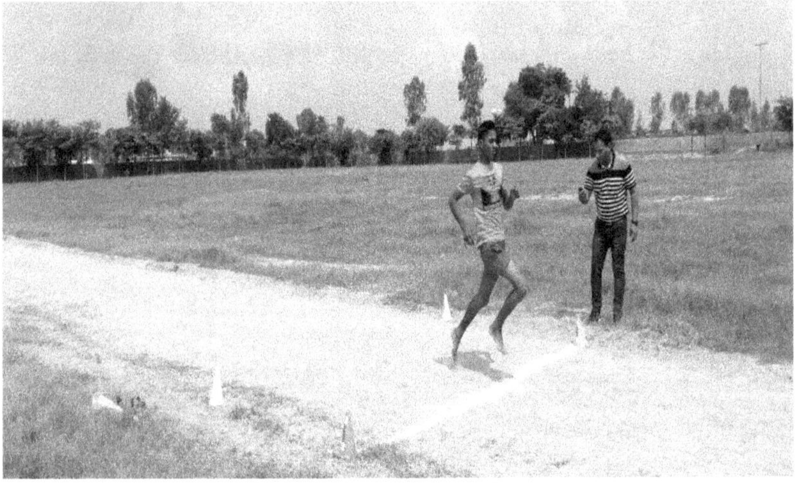

Figure 3.30 50mts. Dash running test

STRENGTH (STANDING BROAD JUMP)

Objective: To measure the strength of an individual

Facilities and Equipments required: Jumping pit, Marking powder and measuring tape.

Procedure and Scoring: The subject was made to stand behind the take off line, which was marked on the back of the jumping pit, with feet apart. Before jumping, the examinee should swing the arm backward and bent the knees. To execute the jump, the subject had to swing the arms forward, extend the knees, and jump forward as for as possible, attempting to land on the feet and fall forward instead of backward, if balance is lost. Three trials were taken and the best performance was recorded as the final score. Measurements were taken in meters to the nearest centimeter. The best performance was recorded as the score.

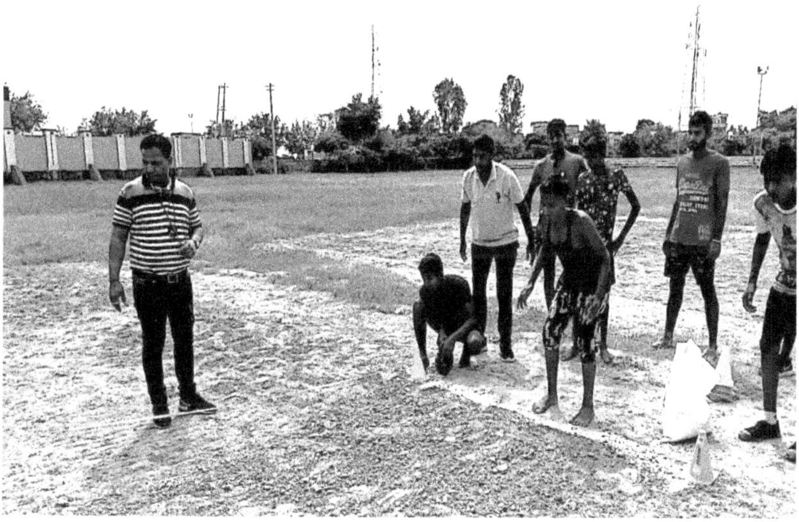

Figure 3.31 Broad jump tests

AGILITY (SHUTTLE RUN)

Objective: To measure agility of the subjects.

Facilities and Equipments required: Measuring tape, clapper and stopwatches.

Procedures and Scoring: Two parallel lines were marked on the floor 10 yards apart. The two wooden blocks were placed behind one of the lines. The subject was asked to start from behind the other line, On the signal ready go, the timer started the watch and the subject ran towards the blocks, picked up one block, ran back to the starting line, placed the block behind the starting line, ran back and picked up the second block to be carried back across the starting line. As soon as the second block was placed on the ground the timer stopped the watch and recorded the time. Two trails were allowed to each subject with some rest in between. The time of the better of the two trails were recorded in seconds as the score of the test item.

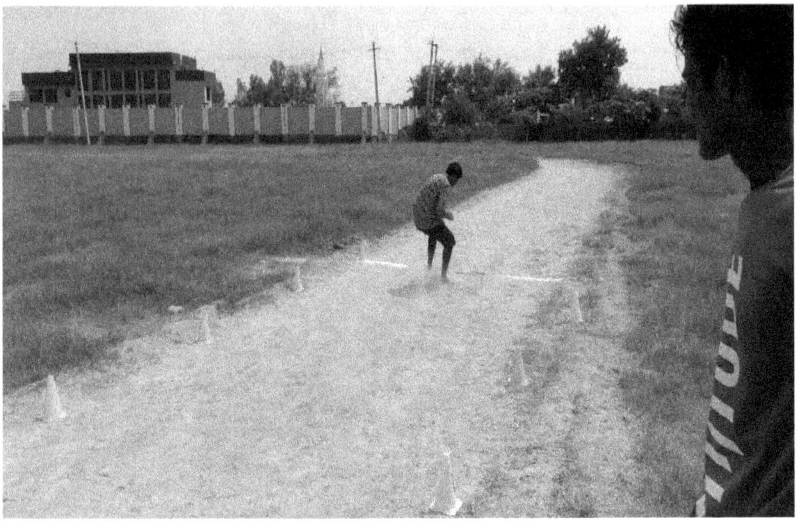

Figure 3.32 (SHUTTLE RUN) test

FLEXIBILITY (SIT AND REACH)

Objective: To measure the flexibility level of the subject.

Facilities and Equipments required: Measuring tape, scales and flexibility bench.

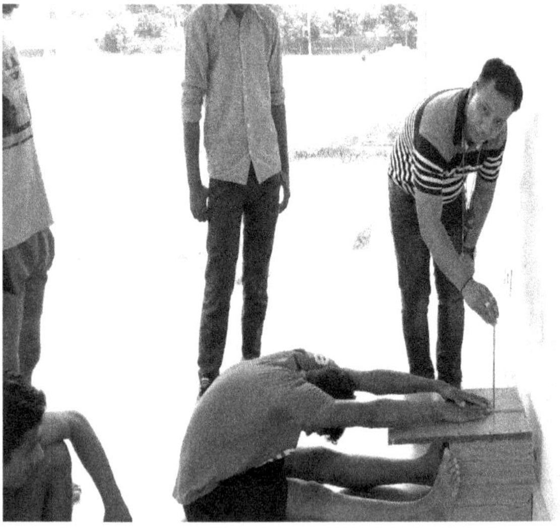

Figure 3.33 (SIT AND REACH) test

Procedure and Scoring: The subject sat on the floor, legs extended and feet flat against a flexibility measurement bench (box with a ruler attached). The trunk was then flexed and the fingers extended along the scale where they were held for a period of 3 seconds. The legs remained extended at the knees throughout the test. The score was recorded in centimeters as either a plus if distances beyond the feet were recorded or a minus if the subject could not reach his feet. Three trials were given after the subject had thoroughly warmed-up.

ENDURANCE (12 MINUTES RUN/ WALK)

Objective: To measure endurance of the subjects

Facilities and Equipments required: Measuring tape, clapper, cones and stopwatches.

Procedures and Scoring: A 400 m track was marked with the help of cones, which was to be 20 meters apart. From starting line on signal, the subjects were started running continuously. At the end of the time allotted for the respective tests, a signal was given where subjects stopped running. The distance covered by individuals in 12 minutes was their individual score. If any subject stopped running or started walking, his timing was not considered as the score. In those cases, one more trial was given.

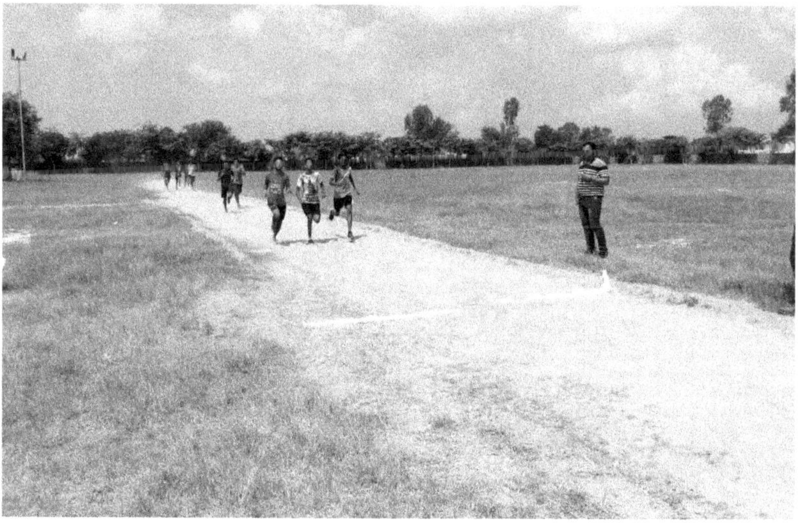

Figure 3.34 (12Minutes walk/run) test

PHYSIOLOGICAL VARIABLES

BLOOD PRESSURE (SYSTOLIC AND DIASTOLIC)

Objective of the test -To measure the blood pressure

Instrument – Sphygmomanometer and stethoscope.

Procedure

The blood pressure was measured to take with the subject in the sitting position, the fore arm was kept straight in a relax position on the table. The pressure cuff was wrapped around the arm evenly. The stethoscope receiver was placed firmly over the bronchial artery. The cuff was inflated until the artery fully pressed so that no pulse beat would hear. Air was slowly released by opening the air valve and the systolic stroke of the heart sent the blood spurt into the artery and the peak of the systolic stroke the first pulse beat become audible at which instant the reading of the mercury was recorded in millimeter. With the gradual release of the air the pulse beat became more and more audible and then sound became muffle and then disappeared. This indicated blood pressure at the diastolic stage and the reading was recorded in millimeter.

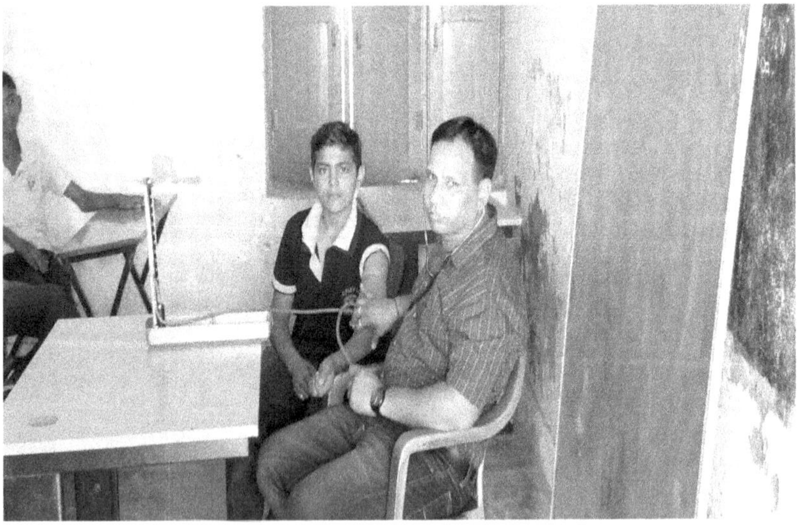

Figure 3.35 Blood pressure measurements

RESTING HEART RATE

Objective of the test

To find out the resting heart rate.

Instrument - A stop watch

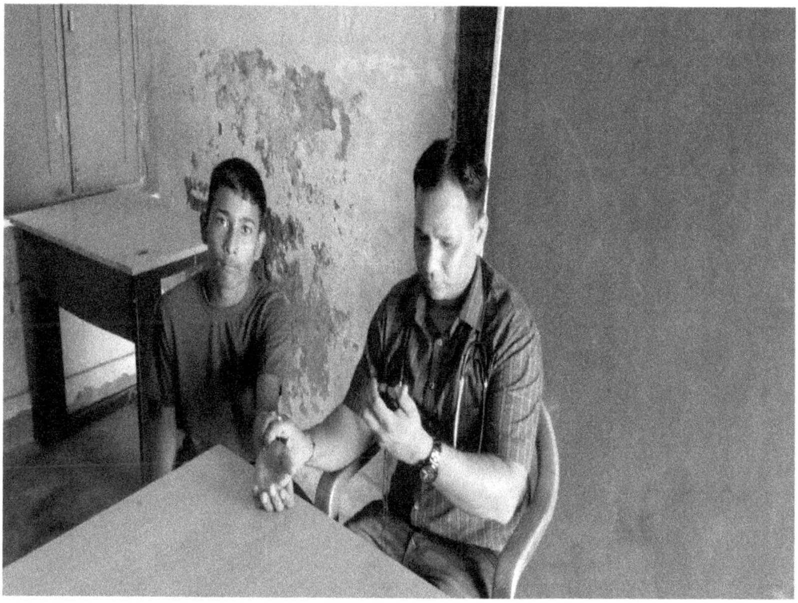

Figure 3.36 Resting heart rate test

Procedure

The pulse rate of the subject was recorded in the sitting position. Before taking the normal pulse rate subject was asked to relax in the sitting position for 20 minutes. The pulse rate was taken at the wrist in such a manner that palpitation was clearly felt by the finger tips. The measurement of palpitation was counted for one minute

BREATH HOLDING TIME

Objective of the test

To find out the ability of the subject to hold his breath for maximum duration

Instrument: A stop watch.

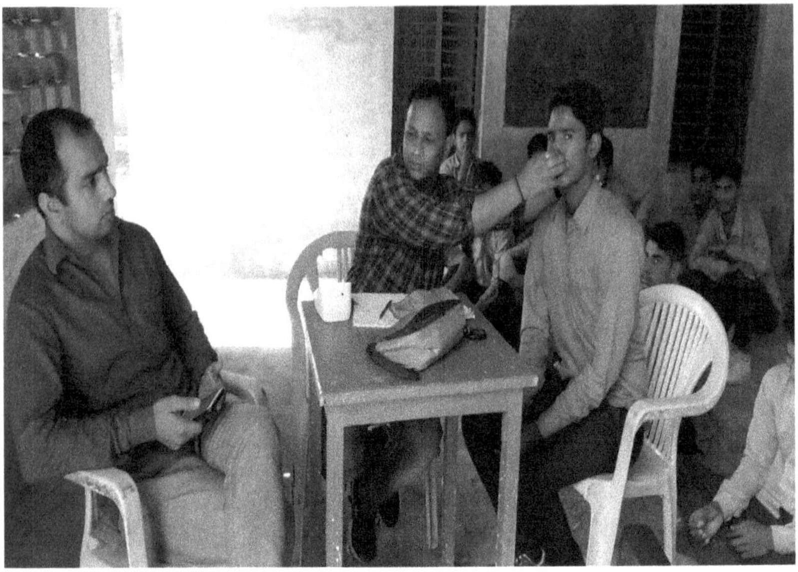

Figure 3.37 Breath holding time test

Procedure:

The test consists of a voluntary force inhalation and holding the breath as long as possible without inhaling or exhaling after holding the breath. Two trials were permitted for each subject and the best time was recorded.

Scoring: - The best of two breath holding time was recorded in seconds as score.

HAEMATOLOGICAL VARIABLES (COMPLETE BLOOD COUNT TEST)

Objective of the test: - To know the concentration of blood cellular parts which was used as haematilogical variables of study:

1. White blood cell
2. Red blood cell
3. Haemoglobin
4. Platelets count

Instrument: Antiseptic lotion, tourniquet, needle and syringes, blood sample tubes and automated hematology analyzer.

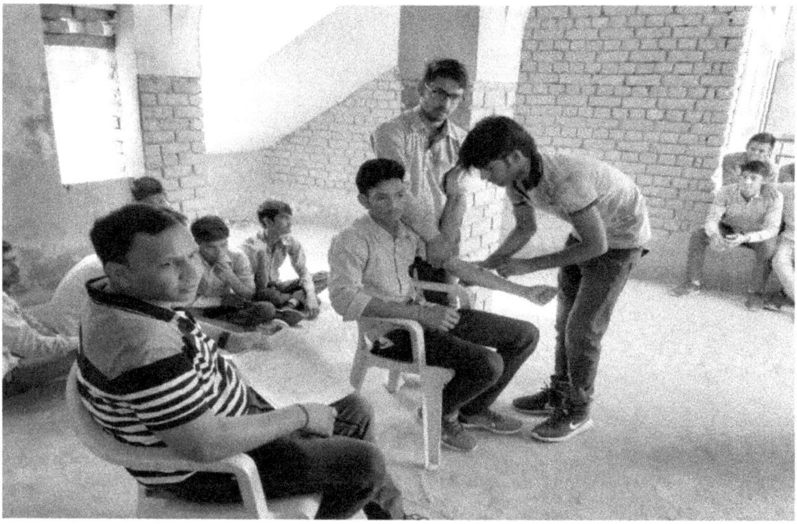

Figure 3.38 Blood Sampling for CBC Test.

Procedure:

A complete blood count (CBC) is also known as a full blood count. It is a medical laboratory test that provide information about the cells in a person`s blood. Blood sample of all the subjects for the haematological variables concentration was collected with the help of a qualified medical lab technician. He draws blood from a vein from the inside of elbow of the subjects. He cleans skin with an antiseptic wipe. Place tourniquet around upper arm to help the vein swell with blood. Collect blood sample with the help of needle and syringe. Cover the area with a bandage to stop any bleeding. Blood sample was taken from the subjects in fasting condition in the morning. All blood samples sent the medical laboratory. Fully automated hematology analyzer was used to find out the concentration of haematological variables.

COLLECTION OF DATA:

The data were collected two times in the study. Asana training (AT), Pranayama training (PT) and Asana & Pranayama Combined training (APT) were conducted for a period of twelve weeks. Observation for test was collected prior to treatment and at the end of twelve weeks of trainings. Essential instructions were given to the subjects. Before the administration of tests tester gave demonstration and information about each test items and also given one trial to subjects to make them acquainted with the testing method. The tests were organized to collect the data of physical fitness, physiological and haematological variables at the time which was practical and suitable to organization and the subjects with the goal that their standard time table not to be disturb.

STATISTICAL PROCEDURE:

The study sample was checked for homogeneity by Levene's test between four groups during pre-test. To find out the significant effects of training each group was assessed and compared on the basis of pre-test and post-test with paired sample t-test. To identify most effective training programme for each and every parameter regarding physical fitness, physiological and hematological well being, respective groups were evaluated using Uni-variate analysis of covariance (ANCOVA). The analysis of covariance was next step of one way analysis of variance (ANOVA) which included the covariate and used to eliminate the effects of co-variance of a third factor on the dependent variable. The groups interaction effects were also observed to analyze the effects of given training between the groups. The level was significance was 95% for all inferential statistics.

SUMMARY OF THE CHAPTER:

This chapter presented and defined the methodology used for this study. Design of the study selection of subjects, selection of variables, selection of tests, criterion measures, reliability of data, instrumental reliability, tester`s reliability, pilot study, training programmes, administration of tests, collection of data and statistical procedure have been explained in detail. This chapter shows that how the choice of the design of the study and selected methods of research suited to answering the research problem. In the next chapter „Result and Discussion" analysis and interpretation of the data was presented. Comments on results and what they mean also have been explained.

CHAPTER – IV

ANALYSIS OF THE DATA, RESULTS AND DISCUSSION

Data analysis and results of the study:

Exercise, in any form is important for the body to keep it in shape and improving endurance. Ancient Indians had recognised the role of yoga for creating balance, attainment of strength, improving flexibility and relaxing the body through postures, simple movements and breathing patterns. Now the whole world is trying to understand yoga and practising it.

The present chapter has been planned to present the analysis and interpretation of present research work. As per the formulated objectives the present study has been designed to investigate the effects of hatha yoga on physical fitness, physiological and hematological variables of school level students respectively. For accomplishing the study four groups were randomly assigned. Out of four groups, Group A was assigned yoga asanas training, group B was subjected to pranayamas training and group C was yoga asanas and pranayamas combination for the duration of 12 weeks with five days per week while group D was monitored as control group. The control group was not participated in any training programme.

To find out the significant effects of training each group was assessed and compared on the basis of pre-test and post-test with paired sample t-test. To identify most effective training programme for each and every parameter regarding physical fitness, physiological and hematological well being, respective groups were evaluated using one way analysis of covariance (ANCOVA). The analysis of covariance was next step of one way analysis of variance (ANOVA) which included the covariate and used to eliminate the effects of co-variance of a third factor on the dependent variable. The groups interaction effects were also observed to analyze the effects of given training between the groups. The level was significance was 95% for all inferential statistics. The obtained data was analyzed and computed with the help of SPSS (Statistical Package for Social Science) version 20.0 which already check the normality through the Levene's test of equality of Error Variance.

SECTION – I ANALYSIS OF PHYSICAL FITNESS PARAMETERS:

For, Objectives:

1. To ascertain the effects of asana training, pranayama training and asana & pranayama combined training on physical fitness variables of their respective group.
2. To find out that which training has better effects on physical fitness variables within asana training, pranayama training and asana & pranayama combined training.

(Null Hypotheses):

1. There would be no significant difference in physical fitness variables on yoga asana group, pranayama group and asana & pranayama combined group due to their respective hatha yoga trainings.
2. It was hypothesized that asana training, pranayama training and asana & pranayama combined training equally effects the physical fitness variables of their respective group.

1. Speed:

Speed of students was assessed with 50m dash run. The time taken by them was noted in seconds.

Table 4.1 Mean speed for 50 m dash (Second) run among groups in pre-test

Group	N	Mean	Std. Deviation	Levene Statistic	p-value
Group A	25	8.12	0.73	1.749	0.162^{NS}
Group B	25	8.44	1.13		
Group C	25	8.12	0.58		
Group D	25	8.17	0.74		
Total	100	8.21	0.82		

NS- Non-Significant ($p>0.05$)

The Table 4.1 depicts the descriptive statistics of groups in terms of mean and standard deviation during pre-test. Mean and standard deviation during pre-test of Group A(Yoga Asana) was 8.12 ± 0.73, for Group B(Pranayama) group was 8.44 ±

1.13, for Group C(Asana and Pranayama Mixed Group) was 8.12 ± 0.58 and mean and Standard Deviation of Group D(Control group) was 8.17 ± 0.74 respectively. Total 100 students took average 8.21 ± 0.82 seconds for 50 m dash run. It was taken into notice that Homogeneity of Variances was not significant(0.162; p>0.05) according to Levene Statistic(1.749) showing the homogeneity among students from various groups while performing 50 m dash.

The table 4.2 shows the pre and post test comparison for speed through 50 mts dash. In group A, pre test mean (M- 8.12) was higher than post test mean (M-7.65). The pre test SD was 0.73 and post test SD was 0.72. The mean difference and t value were 0.474 and 9.189 respectively. The p value came out to be significant (p-0.000). In group B, pre test mean (M- 8.44) was slightly higher than post test mean (M- 8.12). The mean difference and t value were 0.320 and 6.964 respectively. The p value came out to be significant (p- 0.000). Pre test mean was 8.12 and post test mean was 7.62 for group C. The t value was 8.659. The p value was significant (p- 0.000). In Group D, pre test mean (M- 8.17) was higher than post test mean (M- 8.11). Pre test SD was 0.74 and post test SD was 0.76.

Table 4.2 : Pre and post-test comparison for speed through 50 mts dash (seconds)

Group		N	Mean	SD	Mean difference	t	Df	p-value
Group A	Pre Test	25	8.12	0.73	0.474	9.189	24	0.000^{S}
	Post Test	25	7.65	0.72				
Group B	Pre Test	25	8.44	1.13	0.320	6.964		0.000^{S}
	Post Test	25	8.12	1.09				
Group C	Pre Test	25	8.12	0.58	0.502	8.659		0.000^{S}
	Post Test	25	7.62	0.56				
Group D	Pre Test	25	8.17	0.74	0.066	1.709		0.100^{NS}
	Post Test	25	8.11	0.76				

S- Significant (p<0.05) NS- Non-Significant (p>0.05)

The Mean difference and t value were 0.066 and 1.709 respectively. The p-value was statistically non-significant (p- 0.100). Although both the training programmes(Yoga asana and Pranayama) significantly decreased the time for 50 mts dash but combination of both was found most effective with maximum mean difference(0.502) compared to pre-test. No specific training group (control) failed to bring significant change in post test than pre-test.

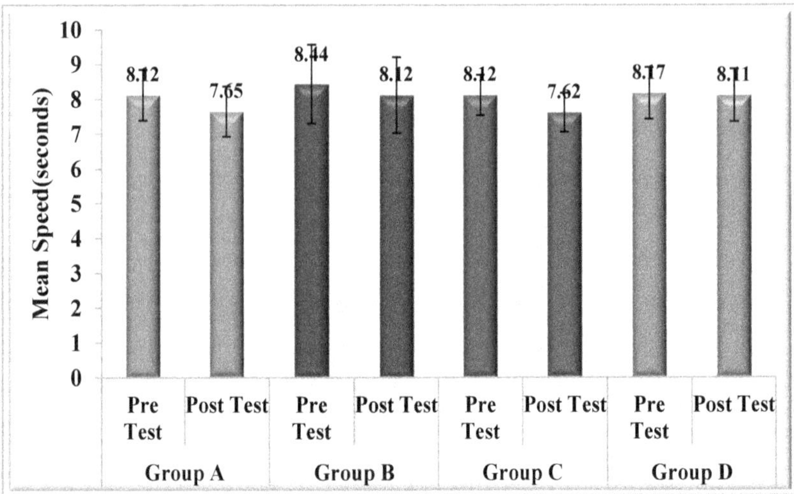

Figure 4.1: Mean speed for 50 Meter Dash Run in pre-test and post-test among various groups

Mean speed for the different groups in terms of 50 mts dash is represented in the graph. In group A, pre test mean was 8.12 and post test mean was 7.65. SD for pre test was 0.73 and for post test was 0.72. In group B, mean in pre test was 8.44 and post test was 8.12. During pre test, SD was 1.13 and during post test, SD was 1.09. Mean in pre test was found to be 8.12 and in post test was 7.62 in group C. SD was 0.58 during pre test and 0.56 during post test. Mean during pre test was 8.17 and post test was 8.11 for Group D. SD was 0.74 during pre test and 0.76 during post test.

Table 4.3 Descriptive Statistics of Groups without Adjustment of Mean speed

Dependent Variable : Speed(50m dash run(Seconds))			
Group	**Mean**	**Std. Deviation**	**N**
Group A	7.65	0.72	25
Group B	8.12	1.09	25
Group C	7.62	0.56	25
Group D	8.11	0.76	25
Total	**7.87**	**0.83**	**100**

The Table 4.3 depicts the descriptive statistics for speed(50m dash run) during post-test without adjusted covariate. It was noticed that mean and standard deviation of post-test for Group A(Yoga Asana) was 7.65 ± 0.72, for Group B(Pranayama) group was 8.12 ± 1.09, for Group C(Asana and Pranayama Mixed Group) was 7.62 ± 0.56 and mean and Standard Deviation of Group D(Control group) was 8.11 ± 0.76 respectively. Mean speed of total hundred students was recorded as 7.87 ± 0.83.

Table 4.4 Levene's Test of Equality of Error Variances

Dependent Variable: Speed(50m dash run(Seconds))			
F	**df1**	**df2**	**Sig.**
0.691	3	96	0.560^{NS}

NS- Non-Significant(p>0.05)

The Table 4.4 illustrates the equality of variance among the groups. The value of $F_{3,96}$ = 0.691 which is not significant at 0.05 level of Alpha.

Table 4.5 Analysis of Covariance for Post Intervention speed (50 Meter Dash run)

Dependent Variable: Speed(50m dash run(Seconds))						
Source	**Type III Sum of Squares**	**df**	**Mean Square**	**F**	**Sig.**	**Partial Eta Squared**
Corrected Model	63.791	4	15.948	271.462	0.000	0.920
Intercept	0.020	1	0.020	0.339	0.562	0.004
Fify mts. dash(pre)	58.012	1	58.012	987.476	0.000	0.912
Group	3.051	3	1.017	17.309	0.000^{S}	0.353
Error	5.581	95	0.059			
Total	6276.134	100				
Corrected Total	69.372	99				
a. R Squared = .920 (Adjusted R Squared = .916)						

S- Significant(p<0.05)

The table 4.5 reveals whether the different interventions were statistically considerable having adjusted for covariate. It was observed that the calculated value of F for group's interaction was 17.309 which were statistically significant at 0.05 level of alpha. The F value illustrate significant difference in post intervention of 50 meter dash run between the selected groups after adjusted the covariate pretest of respective variable. Therefore, the adjusted mean significantly varies among the groups after covariate the pretest. The relationship of various training programmes on the speed of students was seen very strong with regression ($R^2 = 0.920$).

Table 4.6: Post Hoc Analysis for Speed 50 Meter Dash run (Seconds)

(I) GROUPS	(J) GROUPS	Mean Difference (I-J)	Std. Error	p-value
Group A(Yoga Asana)	Group B	-0.173	0.069	0.014^{S}
	Group C	0.028	0.069	0.679^{NS}
	Group D	-0.411	0.069	0.000^{S}
Group B(Pranayama)	Group C	0.201	0.069	0.005^{S}
	Group D	-0.238	0.069	0.001^{S}
Group C (Asana and Pranayama Mixed Group)	Group D	-0.439	0.069	0.000^{S}

The table 4.6 shows the pair-wise comparison of mean scores among four groups namely Yoga Asana Group A, Pranayama Group B, Asana and pranayama mixed Group C and Control group. The mean difference between Group A(Yoga Asana) and Group B(Pranayama) was -0.173 which was significant at .05 level of alpha. The mean difference with Group C(mixed group) was 0.028 which was not significant and mean difference with control group was -0.411 which was highly significant at .05 level of alpha. Mean difference of Group B compared to Group C(Pranayama and Mixed Group) was 0.201 and with control group was -0.238 and both were statistically significant. The Mean difference of Group C(Mixed Group) with Group D(Control Group) was -0.439 and significance value is lower than .05. Therefore Group C(mixed group) shows higher mean difference with Group D(control group).

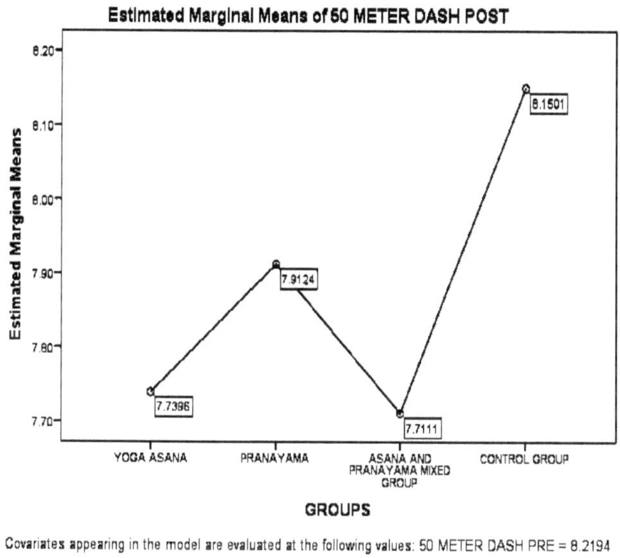

Figure 4.2 Mean Plot for speed (50 Meter Dash Run) during post test

The above figure 4.2 shows adjusted means in post-test for pre-test in all four groups. It was seen that mean time (M-7.71 seconds) was least for Group C (Asana and Pranayama mixed group) proving mixed training best for increasing speed.

2. Strength:

The researcher had considered broad jump as a measure of strength. The unit for broad jump was meter.

Table 4.7 Average strength during broad jump (meter) by groups in pre-test

GROUP	N	Mean	Std. Deviation	Levene Statistic	p-value
Group A	25	1.70	0.20	0.572	0.635^{NS}
Group B	25	1.77	0.17		
Group C	25	1.80	0.22		
Group D	25	1.79	0.22		
Total	100	1.77	0.20		

In pre-test average strength during standing broad jump of students in various groups has been depicted in Table 4.7. In strength test Group A had mean 1.70 ± 0.20, Group

B 1.77 ± 0.17, Group C 1.80 ± 0.22 and Group D 1.79 ± 0.22 respectively. The mean broad jump of 100 students was 1.77 ± 0.20 meter. Homogeneity of Variances was found not significant (0.635; $p>0.05$) according to Levene Statistic (0.572).

Table 4.8 : Pre and post-test comparison for strength during Broad jump (mts)

Group		N	Mean	SD	Mean difference	t	Df	p-value
Group A	Pre Test	25	1.70	0.20	-0.157	-12.219	24	0.000^{S}
	Post Test	25	1.86	0.17				
Group B	Pre Test	25	1.77	0.17	-0.065	-5.590		0.000^{S}
	Post Test	25	1.84	0.17				
Group C	Pre Test	25	1.80	0.22	-0.096	-9.717		0.000^{S}
	Post Test	25	1.90	0.23				
Group D	Pre Test	25	1.79	0.22	-0.009	-1.208		0.239^{NS}
	Post Test	25	1.80	0.22				

S- Significant ($p<0.05$)   NS- Non-Significant ($p>0.05$)

The Table 4.8 represents the pre and post test comparison for strength during broad jump. In group A, pre test mean (M- 1.70) was lower than post test mean (M-1.86). The pre test SD was 0.20 and post test SD was 0.17. The mean difference and t value were -0.157 and -12.219 respectively. The p value came out to be significant (p-0.000). Pre test mean (M- 1.77) was lower than post test mean (M- 1.84). The SD during both tests was same (SD- 0.17). Pre test mean was 1.80 and post test mean was 1.90 for group C. The t value was -9.717. The p value was statistically significant (p-0.000). In group D, pre test mean (M- 1.79) and post test mean (M- 1.80) was almost same. SD for both groups was 0.22.

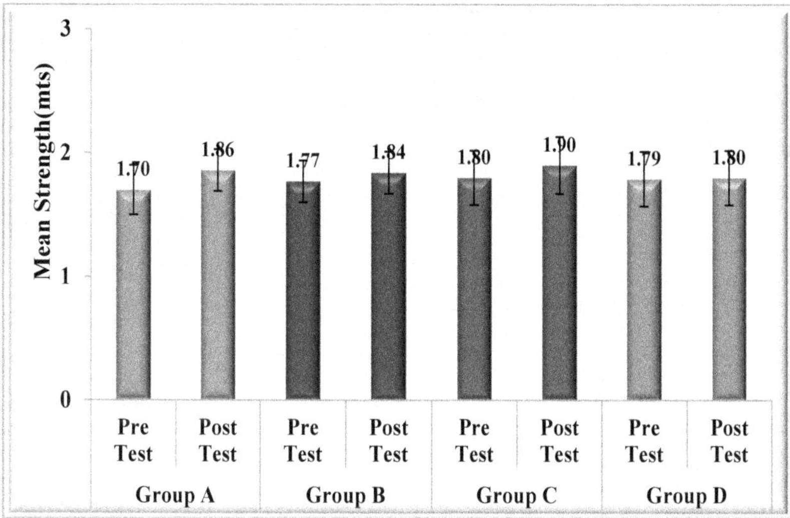

Figure 4.3 : Pre and post test comparison for strength during standing broad jump

Mean strength of different groups in terms of broad jump is represented in the graph. In group A, pre test mean was 1.70 and post test mean was 1.86. SD for pre test was 0.20 and for post test was 0.17. In group B, mean in pre test and post test was 1.77 and 1.84 respectively. SD for both tests was 0.17. Mean in pre test was found to be 1.80 and in post test was 1.90 in group C. SD was 0.22 during pre test and 0.23 during post test. Mean during pre test and post test was 1.79 and 1.80 for group D. SD was 0.22 for both pre test and post test.

Table 4.9 Descriptive Statistics for without Adjusted Mean strength

Dependent Variable: Strength(Standing broad jump(mts))			
Group	**Mean**	**Std. Deviation**	**N**
Group A	1.86	0.17	25
Group B	1.84	0.17	25
Group C	1.90	0.23	25
Group D	1.80	0.22	25
Total	**1.85**	**0.20**	**100**

The Table 4.9 depicts the descriptive statistics in terms of mean and standard deviation without adjusted covariate. It was take into notice that mean and standard deviation of posttest of Group A was 1.86 ± 0.177, for Group B was 1.84±.177, for Group C was 1.90 ± 0.232 and mean and Standard Deviation of Group D was 1.80 ± 0.228 respectively. Total 100 students showed mean 1.85 meter mean strength for standing broad jump.

Table 4.10: Equality of Variance among Groups for Standing Broad Jump

Dependent Variable: Strength(Standing broad jump(mts))			
F	**df1**	**df2**	**Sig.**
0.802	3	96	0.496^{NS}

NS- Non-Significant(p>0.05)

The Table 4.10 illustrates the equality of variance among the groups. The value of $F_{3,96} = 0.802$ which is not significant($p=0.496$; $p>0.05$).

Table 4.11: Analysis of Covariance for Post Intervention Standing Broad Jump

Dependent Variable: Strength(Standing broad jump(mts))						
Source	**Type III Sum of Squares**	**Df**	**Mean Square**	**F**	**Sig.**	**Partial Eta Squared**
Corrected Model	3.922[a]	4	0.981	349.025	0.000	0.936
Intercept	0.036	1	0.036	12.872	0.001	0.119
SBJ_PRE	3.786	1	3.786	1347.518	0.000	0.934
GROUPS	0.268	3	0.089	31.775	0.000^{S}	0.501
Error	0.267	95	0.003			
Total	348.255	100				
Corrected Total	4.189	99				
a. R Squared = .936 (Adjusted R Squared = .934)						

S- Significant(p<0.05)

The table 4.11 reveals that different interventions were statistically considerable having adjusted for covariate. It was observed that the calculated value of F for group's interaction was 31.775 which were statistically significant at 0.05 level of alpha. The F value illustrates significant difference in post intervention strength during Standing Broad Jump between the selected groups after adjusted the covariate pretest. Therefore, the adjusted mean significantly varies among the groups showing strong relationship($R^2 = 0.936$).

Table 4.12: Post-hoc Analysis for Strength (Standing Broad Jump)

(I) GROUPS	(J) GROUPS	Mean Difference (I-J)	Std. Error	p-value
Group A(Yoga Asana)	Group B	0.088	0.015	0.000^S
	Group C	0.056	0.015	0.000^S
	Group D	0.144	0.015	0.000^S
Group B(Pranayama)	Group C	-0.033	0.015	0.032^S
	Group D	0.056	0.015	0.000^S
Group C(Asana and Pranayama Mixed Group)	Group D	0.088	0.015	0.000^S

S- Significant($p<0.05$)

The table 4.12 shows the pairwise comparison of mean strength among four groups Group A(Yoga Asana), Group B(Pranayama), Group C(Asana and pranayama mixed) and Group D(Control). All the paired comparisons showed significant mean differences between groups. Students from Group A showed maximum strength compared to Group B as well as Group C with 0.088 and 0.056 mean difference respectively during post-test which indicates that Asana training(Group A) improved the strength among students more individually as well as combined with Pranayama(Group C).

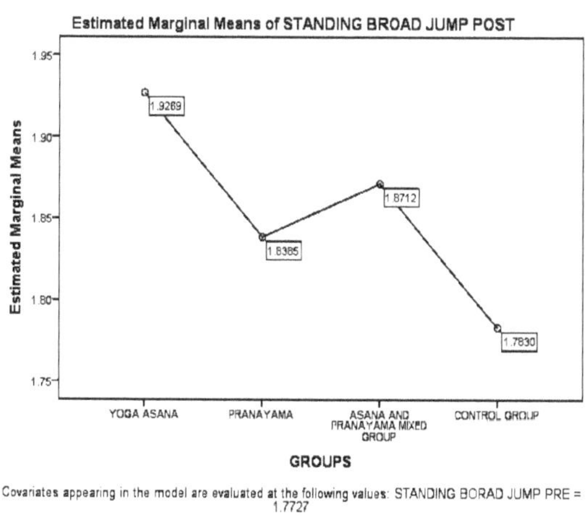

Figure 4.4: Mean Plot for strength (Standing Broad Jump) during post test

The above figure 4.4 shows adjusted means in post-test for pre-test in all four groups. It was seen that mean strength (M-1.92) was maximum for Group A(Asana), followed by mixed group(M-1.87). Asana training individually was found best for strength improvement among students.

3. Agility:

The agility among students was assessed while performing shuttle run. The measuring unit was seconds.

Table 4.13: Average agility while Shuttle Run (seconds) among groups in pre-test

GROUP	N	Mean	Std. Deviation	Levene Statistic	p-value
Group A	25	11.67	0.58	1.033	0.382^{NS}
Group B	25	11.78	0.82		
Group C	25	11.40	0.56		
Group D	25	11.89	0.55		
Total	100	11.69	0.65		

NS- Non-Significant(p>0.05)

In pre-test average agility during Shuttle run of students in various groups has been depicted in Table 4.13. In strength test Group A had mean 11.67 ± 0.58, Group B 11.78 ± 0.82, Group C 11.40 ± 0.56 and Group D 11.89 ± 0.55 respectively. The mean agility of 100 students was 11.69 ± 0.65 seconds. Homogeneity of Variances was found not significant (0.382; p>0.05) according to Levene Statistic (1.033).

Table 4.14: Pre and post-test comparison for agility through Shuttle run (seconds)

Group		N	Mean	SD	Mean difference	t	Df	p-value
Group A	**Pre Test**	25	11.67	0.58	0.669	7.372	24	0.000^{S}
	Post Test	25	11.00	0.61				
Group B	**Pre Test**	25	11.78	0.82	0.680	7.954		0.000^{S}
	Post Test	25	11.10	0.67				
Group C	**Pre Test**	25	11.40	0.56	0.807	7.537		0.000^{S}
	Post Test	25	10.60	0.74				
Group D	**Pre Test**	25	11.89	0.55	-0.063	-1.408		0.172^{NS}
	Post Test	25	11.95	0.69				

S- Significant (p<0.05) NS- Non-Significant (p>0.05)

The table 4.14 shows the pre and post test comparison for shuttle run. In group A, pre test mean (M- 11.67) was higher than post test mean (M-11.00). The pre test SD was 0.58 and post test SD was 0.61. The mean difference and t value were 0.669 and 7.372 respectively. The p value came out to be significant (p- 0.000). In group B, pre test mean was 11.78 and post test mean was 11.10. The mean difference and t value were 0.680 and 7.954 respectively. The p value came out to be significant (p- 0.000). Pre test mean was 11.40 and post test mean was 10.60 for group C. The t value was 7.537. The p value was significant (p- 0.000). In Group D, pre test mean (M- 11.89) was slightly lower than post test mean (M- 11.95). Pre test SD was 0.55 and post test SD was 0.69. The mean difference and t value were -0.063 and -1.408 respectively. The p-value was statistically non-significant (p- 0.172).

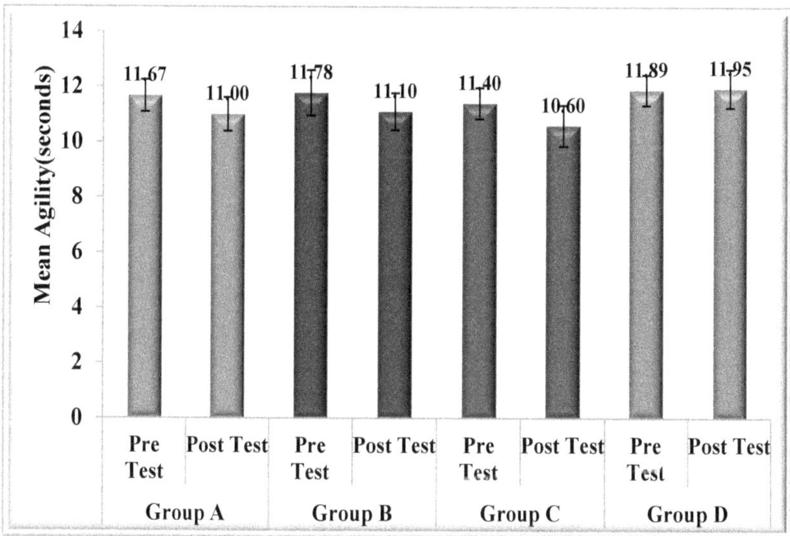

Figure 4.5: Pre and post test comparison for agility through Shuttle run(seconds)

Mean endurance among different groups in terms of shuttle run is represented in the graph Figure 4.5. In group A, with improved agility students completed shuttle run in mean 11.00 seconds during post-test compared to 11.67 in pre-test. Similarly time reduced from average 11.78 seconds to 11.10 in group B. Major change was noticed in Group C with mean 10.60 from 11.40 seconds. Reverse agility was visible among control group where time for shuttle run increased from 11.89 to 11.95.

Table 4.15: Statistics for without Adjusted Mean agility during post-test

Dependent Variable: Agility(Shuttle run (seconds))			
Group	Mean	Std. Deviation	N
Group A	11.00	0.61	25
Group B	11.10	0.67	25
Group C	10.60	0.74	25
Group D	11.95	0.69	25
Total	**11.16**	**0.83**	**100**

The Table 4.15 depicts the descriptive statistics in terms of mean and standard deviation without adjusted covariate. It was noticed that mean and standard deviation in posttest for Group C 10.60 ± 0.74 seconds was minimum and mean agility among Group D 11.95 ± 0.69 was maximum indicating more time taken by control group during shuttle run. The average overall agility of students was calculated as 11.16 ± 0.83.

Table 4.16: Equality of Variance among Groups for Shuttle Run in post-test

Dependent Variable: Agility(Shuttle run(seconds))			
F	df1	df2	p-value
8.327	3	96	0.000[S]

S- Significant($p<0.05$)

The Table 4.16 illustrates the equality of variance among the groups. The value of **F** is 8.327 which is significant at 0.05 level of Alpha. The null hypothesis that there is an equal variance across groups is not accepted for post-test.

Table 4.17: Analysis of Covariance for Post Intervention Agility (Shuttle Run)

Tests of Between-Subjects Effects						
Dependent Variable: Agility(Shuttle run(seconds))						
Source	Type III Sum of Squares	df	Mean Square	F	Sig.	Partial Eta Squared
Corrected Model	55.075[a]	4	13.769	90.448	0.000	0.792
Intercept	1.041	1	1.041	6.836	0.010	0.067
SHUTTLE_RUNPRE	30.787	1	30.787	202.246	0.000	0.680
GROUPS	8.603	3	2.868	18.839	0.000[S]	0.373
Error	14.462	95	0.152			
Total	12542.629	100				
Corrected Total	69.536	99				
a. R Squared = .792 (Adjusted R Squared = .783)						

S- Significant($p<0.05$)

The table 4.17 reveals whether the different interventions were statistically considerable having adjusted for covariate. It was observed that the calculated value of F for group's interaction was 18.839 which were statistically highly significant at 0.05 level of alpha. The F value illustrates significant difference in post intervention agility through shuttle run between the selected groups after adjusted the covariate pretest of respective variable. Therefore, the adjusted mean are significantly varies among the groups after covariate the pretest. Group and pre-test agility explains 79% variance for post-test among students.

Table 4.18: Post Hoc Analysis for agility, Shuttle run (seconds)

(I) GROUPS	(J) GROUPS	Mean Difference (I-J)	Std. Error	p-value
Group A(Yoga Asana)	Group B	-0.005	0.118	0.965^{NS}
	Group C	0.179	0.119	0.138^{NS}
	Group D	-0.765	0.119	0.000^{S}
Group B(Pranayama)	Group C	0.184	0.121	0.131^{NS}
	Group D	-0.760	0.118	0.000^{S}
Group C(Asana and Pranayama Mixed Group)	Group D	-0.944	0.122	0.000^{S}

S- Significant(p<0.05) NS- Non-Significant(p>0.05)

The table 4.18 shows the pairwise comparison of mean agility among four groups : Group A(Yoga Asana), Group B(Pranayama), Group C(Asana and pranayama mixed) and Group D(Control group). The pair-wise mean difference showed that Control group was significantly below in terms of agility than all three training groups.

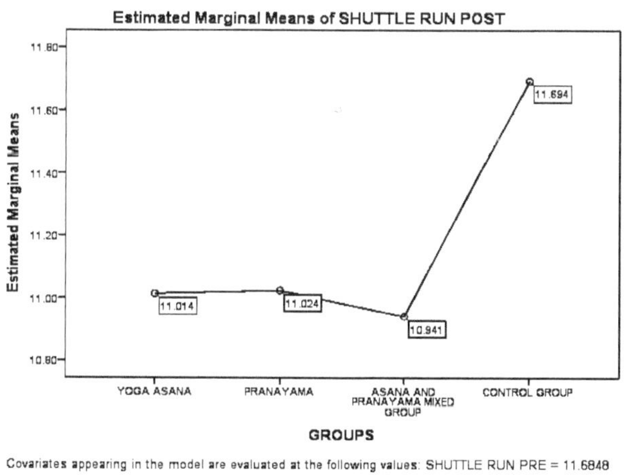

Figure 4.6 : Mean Plot for agility(Shuttle Run(seconds) during post-test

It can be seen in Figure 4.6, that during post-test adjusted mean agility of Group C(mean 10.94) was minimum i.e. Group students took minimum time for shuttle run compared to all other groups advocating Yoga asana and Pranayama mixed training for improving agility.

4. Flexibility:

Among physical fitness parameter to assess the flexibility of students, researcher had conducted sit and reach test using measuring unit as centimeter.

Table 4.19 : Average flexibility for sit and reach(cm.) among groups in pre-test

GROUP	N	Mean	Std. Deviation	Levene Statistic	p-value
Group A	25	7.41	4.19		
Group B	25	8.04	3.19		
Group C	25	7.56	3.95	1.033	0.382^{NS}
Group D	25	5.84	3.66		
Total	100	7.21	3.80		

NS- Non-Significant(p>0.05)

Pre-test flexibility among study groups has been shown in Table 4.19. All the groups were found non-significantly(p-0.382; p>0.05) similarly flexible. The Mean flexibility of Group B was maximum(M-8.04) and Group D was minimum(M-5.84) resulting in 7.21 ± 3.80 cm. overall flexibility for sit and reach test.

Table 4.20 : Pre and post-test comparison of Flexibility(Sit and reach(cm))

Group		N	Mean	SD	Mean difference	t	df	p-value
Group A	Pre Test	25	7.41	4.19	-2.344	-9.601	24	0.000^{S}
	Post Test	25	9.75	3.97				
Group B	Pre Test	25	8.04	3.19	-1.176	-8.652		0.000^{S}
	Post Test	25	9.22	3.35				
Group C	Pre Test	25	7.56	3.95	-1.976	-14.307		0.000^{S}
	Post Test	25	9.54	3.62				
Group D	Pre Test	25	5.84	3.66	-0.136	-1.332		0.195^{NS}
	Post Test	25	5.97	3.44				

S- Significant (p<0.05) NS- Non-Significant (p>0.05)

Pre and post test comparison for flexibility through sit and reach is shown in the table 4.20. In group A, pre test mean (M- 7.41) was lower than post test mean (M-9.75). The pre test SD was 4.19 and post test SD was 3.97. The mean difference and t value were -2.344 and -9.601 respectively. The p value came out to be highly significant (p- 0.000; p<0.05). In group B, post test sit and reach mean (M- 9.22) was better than pre test mean (M- 8.04). The t value was -8.652. The p value came out to be significant (p- 0.000). Pre test mean 7.56 increased to 9.54 during post test for group C. The t value -14.307 was highly significant (p- 0.000). In Group D, pre test mean (M- 5.84) was lower than post test mean (M- 5.97). The mean difference and t value -0.136 and -1.332 respectively were found non-significant (p- 0.195).

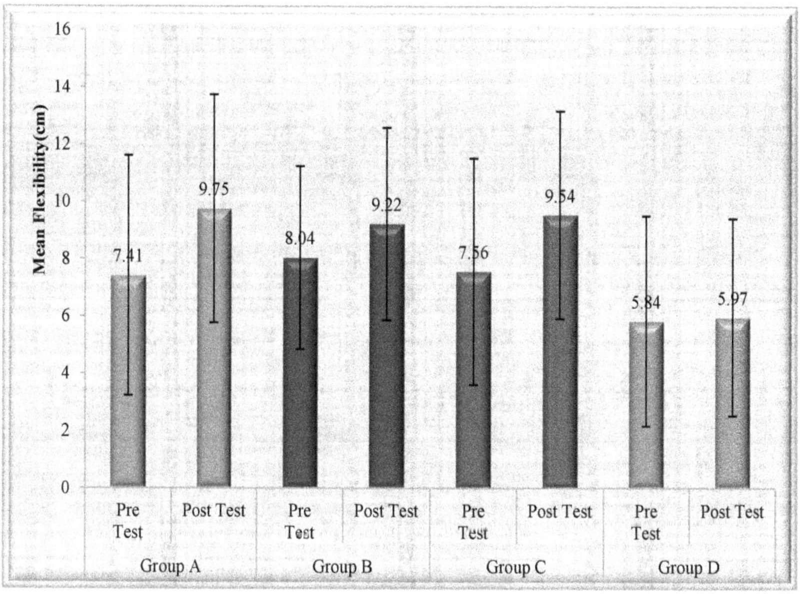

Figure 4.7: Pre and post test comparison for flexibility through Sit and reach (cm)

In Figure 4.7, Mean and SD for the different groups in terms of sit and reach are represented. In group A, pre test mean flexibility (M-7.41) improved up to 9.75cm.in post test. In group B, mean flexibility in pre test was 8.04 which was recorded as 9.22 during post test. Flexibility for pre test was found to be 7.56 and post test 9.54 in group C. Average pre test flexibility was 5.84 and during post test 6.08 among Group D.

Table 4.21 Descriptive Statistics of Flexibility (Sit and Reach (cm.)) without Adjusted Mean

Dependent Variable: Flexibility(Sit and Reach(cm.))			
Group	N	Mean	Std. Deviation
Group A	25	9.75	3.97
Group B	25	9.22	3.35
Group C	25	9.54	3.62
Group D	25	5.97	3.44
Total	100	8.62	3.87

The Table 4.21 depicts the descriptive statistics related to post-test flexibility among students without adjusted covariate. Post-test flexibility of Group A(Yoga Asana) 9.75 ± 3.97 was maximum, followed by Group C(Asana and Pranayama Mixed) 9.54 ± 3.62 where Group B(Pranayama) had mean flexibility as 9.22 ± 3.35. Group D(Control) students were found least flexible having mean 5.97 ± 3.44 in post-test.

Table 4.22 Equality of Variances among Groups regarding Flexibility (Sit and Reach (cm.))

Dependent Variable: Flexibility(Sit and Reach(cm.))			
F	df1	df2	p-value
8.010	3	96	0.000[S]

S- Significant($p<0.05$)

Equality of variance in Table 4.22 was observed highly significantly different among all study groups . The value $\mathbf{F_{3,96}}$ = 8.010 rejected null hypothesis with unequal variance across groups in post-test.

Table 4.23 : Analysis of Covariance among Groups for Post Intervention Flexibility (Sit and Reach(cm.))

Dependent Variable: Flexibility(Sit and Reach(cm.))						
Source	**Type III Sum of Squares**	**Df**	**Mean Square**	**F**	**Sig.**	**Partial Eta Squared**
Corrected Model	1428.380[a]	4	357.095	578.487	0.000	0.961
Intercept	73.614	1	73.614	119.253	0.000	0.557
SIT_AND_REACH_PRE	1191.070	1	1191.070	1929.512	0.000	0.953
GROUPS	76.479	3	25.493	41.298	0.000[S]	0.566
Error	58.643	95	0.617			
Total	8924.360	100				
Corrected Total	1487.022	99				
a. R Squared = .961 (Adjusted R Squared = .959)						

S- Significant ($p<0.05$)

The table 4.23 reveals whether the different interventions were statistically considerable having adjusted for covariate. It was observed that the calculated value of F for group's interaction was 41.298 which were statistically significant($p=0.000$; $p<0.05$). The F value illustrated significant difference in post intervention of sit and reach between the selected groups after adjusted the covariate pretest of respective variable. Therefore, the adjusted mean are significantly varies among the groups after covariate the pretest. Strong 96% variation in post-test flexibility was explained by relationship with group and pre-test flexibility.

Table 4.24 : Post Hoc Analysis for Flexibility(Sit and Reach(cm)) during post-test

(I) GROUPS	(J) GROUPS	Mean Difference (I-J)	Std. Error	p-value
Group A(Yoga Asana)	Group B	1.126	0.223	0.000[S]
	Group C	0.358	0.222	0.111[NS]
	Group D	2.311	0.225	0.000[S]
Group B(Pranayama)	Group C	-0.768	0.222	0.001[S]
	Group D	1.185	0.227	0.000[S]
Group C(Asana and Pranayama Mixed Group)	Group D	1.953	0.225	0.000[S]

S- Significant($p<0.05$) NS- Non-Significant($p>0.05$)

The post-hoc mean difference shown in Table 4.24 was observed significantly higher in Group A than Group B(1.126), and D(2.311) but non-significant(p=0.111; p>005) than Group C(0.358). Students in all three training groups were significantly more flexible compared to control group D.

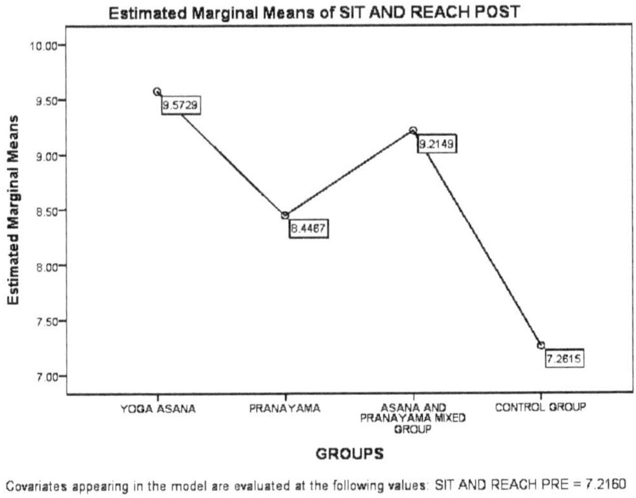

Figure 4.8 : Mean Plot for flexibility(Sit and reach(cm) during post-test

The mean plot for flexibility in Figure 4.8 highlights those students from Group A (Yoga Asana) acquired maximum adjusted mean flexibility (M-9.57) during post-test compared to their counterparts.

5. Endurance:

The researcher had opted cooper run/walk test(12 Minutes).The distance covered in meters during 12 minutes was noted for rating endurance of students.

Table 4.25 : Average pre-test endurance for 12 minute walk/run(meter)

GROUP	N	Mean	Std. Deviation	Levene Statistic	p-value
Group A	25	1852. 80	233.80	2.466	0.067^{NS}
Group B	25	1851.20	236.29		
Group C	25	1956.40	193.49		
Group D	25	1795.20	163.30		
Total	100	1863.90	213.90		

NS- Non-Significant(p>0.05)

The pre-test endurance among students from all groups was found homogenous as shown in Table 4.25. The non-significant p-value(0.067) was calculated while testing for variance. The total students had1863.90 m mean endurance during 12 minute walk and run. Where endurance of Group A(M=1852.80) and Group B(M=1851.20) was almost similar, Group C(M=1956.40) showed maximum and Group D(M=1795.20) minimum Endurance.

Table 4.26 : Pre and post-test comparison of endurance (12 minutes walk run (m))

Group		N	Mean	SD	Mean difference	t	df	p-value
Group A	Pre Test	25	1852.80	233.80	-76.800	-8.609	24	0.000^{S}
	Post Test	25	1929.60	238.68				
Group B	Pre Test	25	1851.20	236.29	-44.000	-6.633		0.000^{S}
	Post Test	25	1895.20	245.51				
Group C	Pre Test	25	1956.40	193.49	-122.800	-9.721		0.000^{S}
	Post Test	25	2079.20	210.90				
Group D	Pre Test	25	1795.20	163.30	8.800	0.447		0.274^{NS}
	Post Test	25	1786.40	157.02				

S- Significant ($p<0.05$) NS- Non-Significant ($p>0.05$)

The Table 4.26, shows the pre and post test comparison for 12 minutes walk run. In group A, pre test mean (M- 1852.80) was lower than post test mean (M-1929.60). The mean difference and t value were -76.800 and -8.609 respectively. The p value came out to be significant (p- 0.000). In group B, students during pre test mean (M-1851.20) covered less distance as compared students during post test (M- 1895.20). The t value was -6.633. The p value came out to be significant (p- 0.000). Pre test mean was 1956.40 and post test mean was 2079.20 for group C. The p-value was significant (p- 0.000). In group D, pre test mean (M- 1795.20) was slightly higher than post test mean (M- 1786.40). The mean difference and t-value were 8.800 and 0.447 respectively. The p-value was statistically non-significant (p- 0.274).

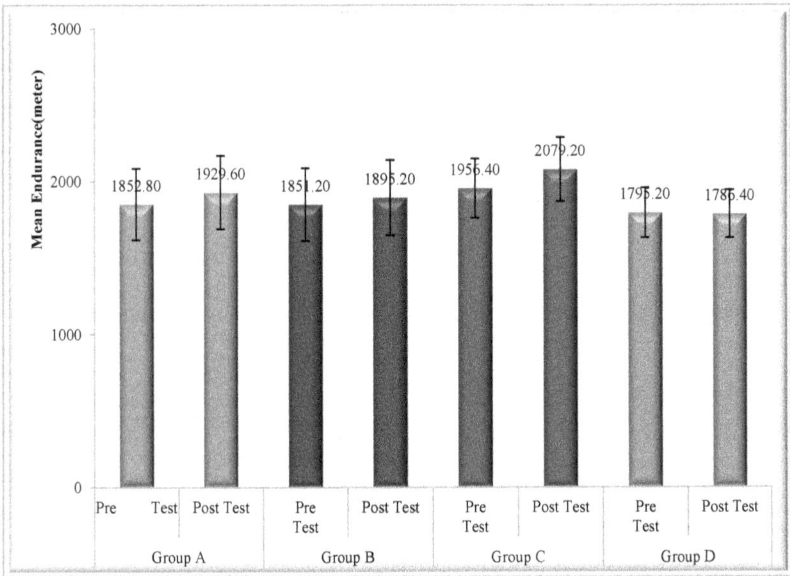

Figure 4.9: Pre and post test comparison for Endurance through 12 minute walk/run(meter)

The above Figure 4.9 shows mean comparison of endurance for different groups in terms of 12 minute walk/run. In group A, pre test mean endurance 1852.80m improved to 1929.60m in post test. In group B, mean in pre test was 1851.20 and post test was 1895.20. Mean pre test was found to be 1956.40 and in post test was 2079.20 in group C. Mean during pre test was 1795.20 and post test was 1786.40 for Group D.

Table 4.27 : Descriptive Statistics of Endurance(12 minutes walk run (m)) without Adjusted Mean

Dependent Variable: Endurance(12 minutes walk run (m))			
Group	**N**	**Mean**	**Std. Deviation**
Group A	25	1929.60	238.68
Group B	25	1895.20	245.51
Group C	25	2079.20	210.90
Group D	25	1786.40	157.02
Total	100	1922.60	237.20

The Table 4.27 depicts the descriptive statistics for endurance without adjusted covariate. The mean and standard deviation in post-test of Group A(Yoga Asana) was 1929.60 ± 238.68, for Group B(Pranayama) was 1895.20 ± 245.51, for Group C(Asana and Pranayama Mixed) was 2079.20 ± 210.90 and mean and Standard Deviation of Group D(Control) was 1922.60 ± 237.20 respectively.

Table 4.28 : Equality of Variance for Endurance(12 minutes walk run (m))

Dependent Variable: Endurance(12 minutes walk run (m))			
F	**df1**	**df2**	**Sig.**
2.227	3	96	0.090^{NS}

NS- Non-Significant (p>0.05)

The Table 4.28 illustrates the equality of variance among the groups. The value of F is 2.227 which is not significant(p=0.090; p>0.05) for endurance during post-test. Hence null hypothesis showing equal variance across groups was accepted.

The table 4.29 depicts that different interventions were statistically considerable having adjusted for covariate. It was observed that the calculated value of F for group's interaction was 23.75 which were statistically significant(p=0.000; p<0.05).

Table 4.29: Analysis of Covariance among Groups for Post Intervention Endurance (12 minutes walk run (m))

Dependent Variable: Endurance(12 minutes walk run (m))						
Source	**Type III Sum of Squares**	**Df**	**Mean Square**	**F**	**Sig.**	**Partial Eta Squared**
Corrected Model	5382755.726[a]	4	1345688.931	682.295	0.000	0.966
Intercept	1771.256	1	1771.256	0.898	0.346	0.009
TWELFTH_MINUTE_RUN_WALK_PRE	4285911.726	1	4285911.726	2173.055	0.000	0.958
GROUPS	140378.393	3	46792.798	23.725	0.000^{NS}	0.428
Error	187368.274	95	1972.298			
Total	375209200.000	100				
Corrected Total	5570124.000	99				
a. R Squared = .966 (Adjusted R Squared = .965)						

The F value illustrate significant difference in post intervention of 12 Minute Run and Walk between the selected groups after adjusted the covariate pretest of respective variable. Therefore, the adjusted mean are significantly varies among the groups after covariate the pretest. Here 96% variation was explained by groups for endurance in post-test.

Table 4.30 : Post Hoc Analysis for Endurance (12 minutes walk run (m)) during post-test

(I) GROUPS	(J) GROUPS	Mean Difference (I-J)	Std. Error	p-value
Group A(Yoga Asana)	Group B	32.778	11.849	0.007^{S}
	Group C	-44.576	12.037	0.000^{S}
	Group D	84.808	11.907	0.000^{S}
Group B(Pranayama)	Group C	-77.354	12.043	0.000^{S}
	Group D	52.030	11.904	0.000^{S}
Group C(Asana and Pranayama Mixed Group)	Group D	129.384	12.300	0.000^{S}

S- Significant($p<0.05$) NS- Non-Significant($p>0.05$)

The Table 4.30 shows the pair-wise comparison of mean endurance among four groups. The mean difference between Group A (Yoga Asana) and Group B(Pranayama) was 32.778 which was significant at .05 level of alpha. All study group were significantly different from each other while considering pair wise comparison for mean endurance.

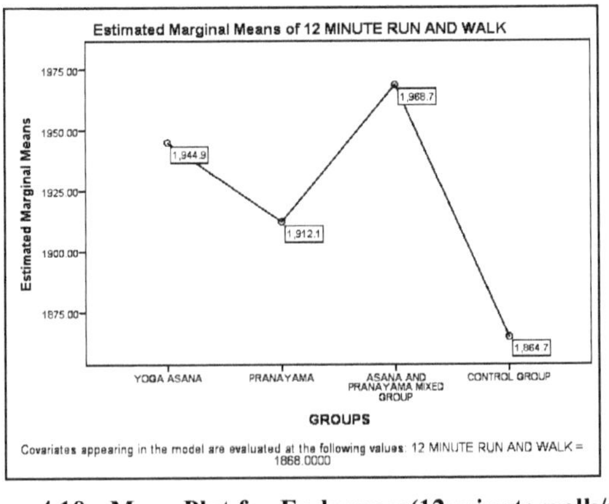

Figure 4.10 : Mean Plot for Endurance(12 minute walk/run (meter) during post-test

Graphical presentation of adjusted mean endurance in Figure 4.10 depicts that Group C(Yoga asana and pranayama mixed) was showing maximum endurance(M=1968.7) during post-test. Even Group A(Yoga asana) and Group B(Pranayama) were better than control group in terms of endurance.

SECTION – II ANALYSIS OF PHYSIOLOGICAL FITNESS VARIABLES

For, Objectives:

1. To ascertain the effects of yoga asana training, pranayama training and asana & pranayama combined training on physiological variables of their respective group.
2. To find out that which training has better effects on physiological variables within asana training, pranayama training and asana & pranayama combined training.

(Null Hypotheses):

1. There would be no significant difference in physiological variables on yoga asana group, pranayama group and asana & pranayama combined group due to their respective hatha yoga trainings.
2. It was hypothesized that asana training, pranayama training and asana & pranayama combined training equally effects the physiological variables of their respective group.

The variables included in the study were-: Systolic Blood pressure, Diastolic Blood Pressure, Heart rate and breath holding capacity.

1. Systolic Blood Pressure:

Among physiological fitness variables most important vital parameter systolic blood pressure was measured in mm/hg.

Table 4.31: Average SBP among groups in pre-test

Group	N	Mean	Std. Deviation	Levene Statistic	p-value
Group A	25	117.64	3.12	0.460	0.711^{NS}
Group B	25	118.68	3.35		
Group C	25	118.96	2.79		
Group D	25	118.64	2.94		
Total	100	118.48	3.05		

NS- Non-Significant(p>0.05)

The above Table 4.31, presented mean systolic blood pressure among students in various groups. The mean SBP of all groups was almost similar. Thus non-significant p=0.711 implied homogeneity between groups during pre-test for SBP. The average SBP of 100 students was 118.48 ± 3.05.

Table 4.32 : Pre and post-test comparison of SBP (mm Hg)

Group		N	Mean	SD	Mean difference	t	df	p-value
Group A	Pre Test	25	117.64	3.12	0.240	0.492	24	0.627^{NS}
	Post Test	25	117.40	2.21				
Group B	Pre Test	25	118.68	3.35	1.160	2.065		0.050^{S}
	Post Test	25	117.52	1.68				
Group C	Pre Test	25	118.96	2.79	1.400	2.425		0.023^{S}
	Post Test	25	117.56	1.87				
Group D	Pre Test	25	118.64	2.94	0.160	0.359		0.723^{NS}
	Post Test	25	118.48	2.36				

S- Significant (p<0.05) NS- Non-Significant (p>0.05)

Pre and post test SBP comparison is showcased in the Table 4.32. In group A, pre test mean (M- 117.64) was slightly higher than post test mean (M- 117.40). The pre test SD was 3.12 and post test SD was 2.21. The t value was 2.065. The p value was non-significant (p- 0.627; p>0.05). In group B, pre test mean was 118.68 and post test mean was 117.52. The t value was 2.065. The p value came out to be borderline significant (p- 0.050). Pre test mean was 118.96 and post test mean was 117.56 for group C. The t value was 2.425. The p value was significant (p- 0.023). In control, pre test mean (M- 118.64) was slightly higher than post test mean (M- 118.48). Pre test SD was 2.94 and post test SD was 2.36. The mean difference and t value were 0.160 and 0.359 respectively. The p-value was statistically non-significant (p- 0.723; p>0.05).

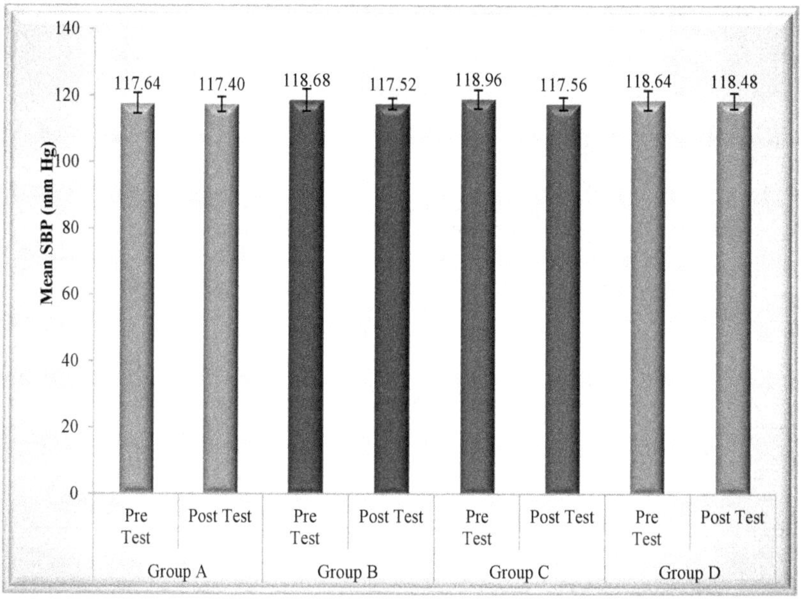

Figure 4.11: Pre and post test comparison for Systolic Blood pressure

Mean and SD for the different groups in terms of SBP is represented in Figure 4.11. In group A, pre test mean was 117.64 and post test mean was 117.40. In group B, mean in pre test was 118.68 and post test was 117.52. Mean in pre test was found to be 118.96 and in post test was 117.56 in group C. Mean during pre test was 118.64 and post test was 118.48 for Control group. As an effect of training SBP of Group B and C were significantly reduced during post-test contrary to Group A and Group D.

Table 4.33 : Descriptive Statistics of Groups without Adjustment for Mean Systolic Blood Pressure

Dependent Variable: Systolic Blood Pressure			
GROUP	**N**	**Mean**	**Std. Deviation**
Group A	25	117.40	2.21
Group B	25	117.52	1.68
Group C	25	117.56	1.87
Group D	25	118.48	2.36
Total	100	117.74	2.06

The Table 4.33 depicts the descriptive statistics in terms of mean and standard deviation without adjusted covariate. It was noticed that mean and standard deviation of post-test in Group A(Yoga Asana) was 117.40 ± 2.21, for Group B(Pranayama) was 117.52 ±1.68, for Group C(Asana and Pranayama Mixed) was 117.56 ± 1.87 and mean and Standard Deviation of Group D(Control) was 118.48± 2.36 respectively. Mean DBP of 100 students was nearly similar to Group A, b and C.

Table 4.34 : Equality of Error Variance among Groups for Systolic Blood Pressure

Dependent Variable: Systolic Blood Pressure			
F	df1	df2	Sig.
0.549	3	96	0.650^{NS}

NS- Non-Significant (p>0.05)

The Table 4.34 illustrates the equality of variance among the groups. The value of F is 0.549 which is not significant at 0.05 level of Alpha. Therefore, the null hypothesis for equal variance across groups was accepted.

The Table 4.35 reveals whether the different interventions were statistically considerable having adjusted for covariate.

Table 4.35: Analysis of Covariance among Groups for Post Intervention Systolic Blood Pressure

Dependent Variable: Systolic Blood Pressure						
Source	Type III Sum of Squares	Df	Mean Square	F	Sig.	Partial Eta Squared
Corrected Model	136.697[a]	4	34.174	11.330	0.000	0.323
Intercept	357.394	1	357.394	118.490	0.000	0.555
SYS_BP_PRE	118.097	1	118.097	39.154	0.000	0.292
GROUPS	16.927	3	5.642	1.871	0.140^{NS}	0.056
Error	286.543	95	3.016			
Total	1386694.000	100				
Corrected Total	423.240	99				

a. R Squared = .323 (Adjusted R Squared = .294)

It was observed that the calculated value of F for group's interaction was 1.871 which was not statistically significant(p=0.140 ; p>0.05). The adjusted means not significantly varied among the groups after covariate the pretest. Only 32% variation in Systolic Blood pressure was explained by groups.

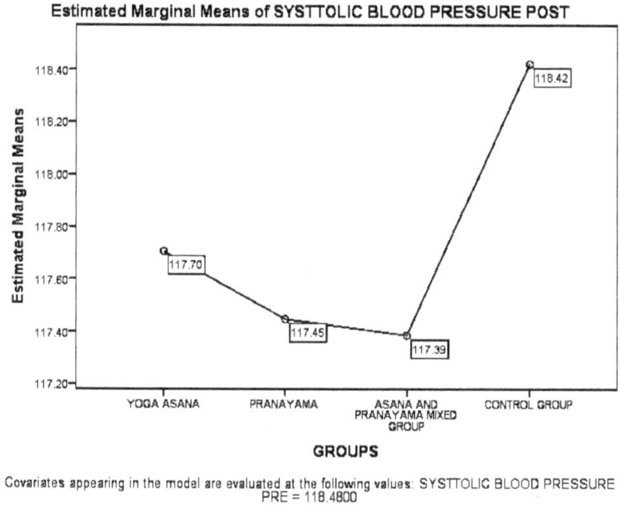

Figure 4.12 : Adjusted Mean Plot for Systolic Blood Pressure during post-test

The current Figure 4.12 illustrates that students of Group C (Asana and Pranayama) were able to reduce their SBP (M=117.39) more easily than other groups.

2. Diastolic Blood pressure:

Diastolic Blood pressure of students in each group was measured in mmHg.

Table 4.36 : Average Diastolic Blood pressure(mmHg) among groups in pre-test

Group	N	Mean	Std. Deviation	Levene Statistic	p-value
Group A	25	77.36	3.55	0.547	0.652^{NS}
Group B	25	77.12	2.90		
Group C	25	77.68	3.07		
Group D	25	76.48	3.02		
Total	100	77.16	3.13		

NS- Non-Significant(p>0.05)

As shown in Table 4.36, The Diastolic Blood Pressure of students during pre-test was homogenous and resulted in non-significant p-value=0.652. Minor mean differences were noticed among students from various groups with mean 77.16 ± 3.13 DBP for all students.

Table 4.37: Pre and post comparison of Diastolic Blood pressure (mm Hg)

Group		N	Mean	SD	Mean difference	t	df	p-value
Group A	Pre Test	25	77.36	3.55	0.360	0.774	24	0.446^{NS}
	Post Test	25	77.00	2.34				
Group B	Pre Test	25	77.12	2.90	1.080	2.119		0.045^{S}
	Post Test	25	76.04	2.22				
Group C	Pre Test	25	77.68	3.07	1.520	2.049		0.052^{NS}
	Post Test	25	76.16	2.47				
Group D	Pre Test	25	76.48	3.02	0.080	0.152		0.880^{NS}
	Post Test	25	76.40	2.44				

S- Significant (p<0.05) NS- Non-Significant (p>0.05)

The Table 4.37 shows the pre and post test comparison for DBP. In group A, pre test mean (M- 77.36) was higher than post test mean (M-77.00). The mean difference and t value were 0.360 and 0.774 respectively. The p value came out to be non-significant (p- 0.446). In group B, mean DBP during pre test was 77.12 and during post test was 76.04. The t value was 2.119. The p value came out to be significant (p- 0.045; p<0.05). Pre test mean was 77.68 and post test mean was 76.16 for group C. The p value was non-significant (p- 0.052). In control group, pre test mean (M- 76.48) was slightly higher than post test mean (M- 76.40). The mean difference and t value were 0.080 and 0.152 respectively. The p-value was statistically non-significant (p- 0.880). All study groups showed decreased DBP in post-test but significant decrease was seen for Group B only. Least decrease was observed among students of control group i.e. Group D.

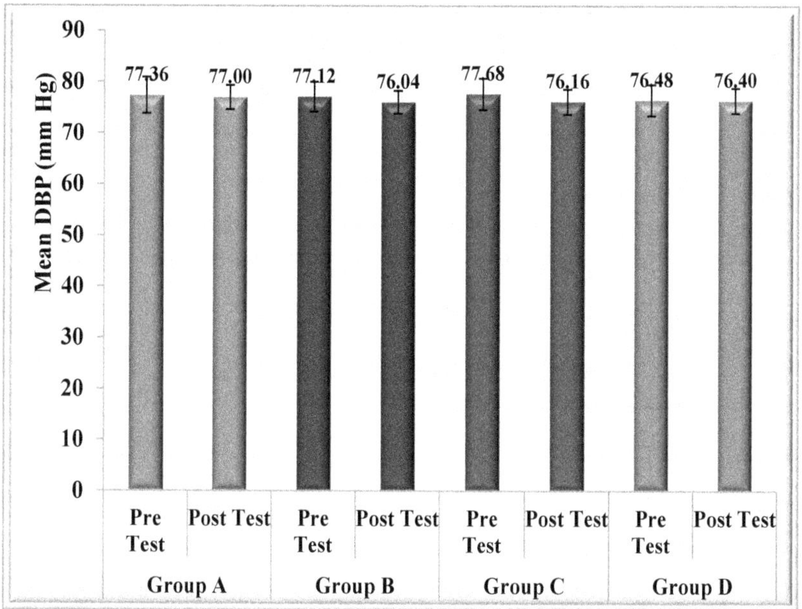

Figure 4.13: Pre and post test comparison for diastolic Blood Pressure

Mean change in DBP is represented in Figure 4.13. In group A, pre test mean DBP was 77.36 and post test mean was 77.00. In group B, mean in pre test was 77.12 and post test was 76.04.. Mean in pre test was found to be 77.68 and in post test was 76.16 in group C. Mean during pre test was 76.48 and post test was 76.40 for Control group. The effect of training could be seen with decreased DBP for Group A, B and C during post-test. Little change was also noticed in Group D.

Table 4.38 : Descriptive Statistics of Diastolic Blood pressure(mm Hg) without Adjusted Mean

Dependent Variable: Diastolic Blood pressure (mm Hg)			
Group	**N**	**Mean**	**Std. Deviation**
Group A	25	77.00	2.34
Group B	25	76.04	2.22
Group C	25	76.16	2.47
Group D	25	76.40	2.44
Total	100	76.40	2.36

The Table 4.38 depicts the descriptive statistics for diastolic blood pressure without adjusted covariate. Mean DBP during post-test of Group A(Yoga Asana) was 77.00 ± 2.34, for Group B(Pranayama) was 76.04 ± 2.22, for Group C(Asana and Pranayama Mixed) was 76.16 ± 2.47 and mean and Standard Deviation of Group D(Control) was 76.40 ± 2.44 respectively.

Table 4.39: Equality of Error Variance among Groups in their Diastolic Blood Pressure

Dependent Variable: Diastolic Blood pressure(mm Hg)			
F	**df1**	**df2**	**Sig.**
3.156	3	96	0.028[S]

NS- Non-Significant (p>0.05)

Tests the null hypothesis that the error variance of the dependent variable is equal across groups. The Table 4.39 illustrates the equality of variance among the groups. The value of F is 3.156 which is significant(p=0.028; p<0.05). Therefore here the null hypothesis having equal variance across groups is not accepted.

The table 4.40 reveals whether the different interventions were statistically considerable having adjusted for covariate.

Table 4.40: Analysis of Covariance among Groups for Post Intervention Diastolic Blood Pressure

Dependent Variable: Diastolic Blood pressure(mm Hg)						
Source	**Type III Sum of Squares**	**Df**	**Mean Square**	**F**	**Sig.**	**Partial Eta Squared**
Corrected Model	147.533[a]	4	36.883	8.578	0.000	0.265
Intercept	360.972	1	360.972	83.954	0.000	0.469
DYSTOLIC_BPPRE	133.853	1	133.853	31.131	0.000	0.247
GROUPS	16.166	3	5.389	1.253	0.295[NS]	0.038
Error	408.467	95	4.300			
Total	584252.000	100				
Corrected Total	556.000	99				
a. R Squared = .265 (Adjusted R Squared = .234)						

It was observed that the calculated value of F for group's interaction was 1.253 which was not statistically significant at 0.05 level of alpha. The F value do not illustrate significant difference in post intervention of Diastolic Blood Pressure between the selected groups after adjusted the covariate pretest of respective variable. The strength of relationship was explained 26% for DBP during post-test.

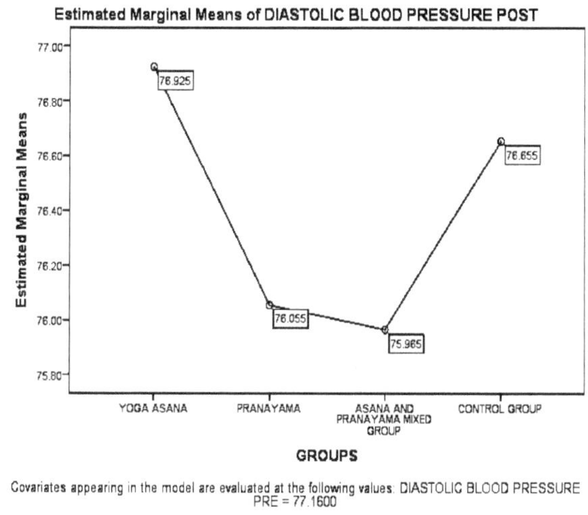

Figure 4.14 : Adjusted Mean Plot for Diastolic Blood Pressure during post-test

The demonstration in Figure 4.14 during post-test highlighted more impact of Yogaasana and pranayama mixed training on DBP of students.

3. Heart rate

Heart rate of student per minute was assessed at resting position.

Table 4.41 : Average Heart rate among groups in pre-test

Group	N	Mean	Std. Deviation	Levene Statistic	p-value
Group A	25	68.72	4.79	0.570	0.636^{NS}
Group B	25	67.84	4.50		
Group C	25	69.60	5.35		
Group D	25	67.92	5.67		
Total	100	68.52	5.07		

NS- Non-Significant(p>0.05)

The pre-test average heart rate, of students in different groups, shown in Table 4.41 was found nearly comparable to each other. All were found homogenous and having non-significant mean difference (p=0.636; p>0.05) The average heart rate of all students was calculated as 68.52 ± 5.07.

Table 4.42: Pre and post comparison of HR (per minute)

Group		N	Mean	SD	Mean difference	t	df	p-value
Group A	Pre Test	25	68.72	4.79	3.200	7.407	24	0.000^{S}
	Post Test	25	65.52	4.33				
Group B	Pre Test	25	67.84	4.50	3.760	7.608		0.000^{S}
	Post Test	25	64.08	3.85				
Group C	Pre Test	25	69.60	5.35	3.600	6.114		0.000^{S}
	Post Test	25	66.00	4.28				
Group D	Pre Test	25	67.92	5.67	-0.480	-0.690		0.497^{NS}
	Post Test	25	68.40	3.95				

S- Significant (p<0.05)   NS- Non-Significant (p>0.05)

Pre and post test comparison for HR is shown in Table 4.42. In group A, heart rate mean was 68.72 during pre test and 65.52 during post test mean. The mean difference and t value were 3.200 and 7.407 respectively. The p value came out to be significant (p- 0.000). In group B, post test heart rate mean (M- 67.84) was better than pre test heart rate mean (M- 64.08). The t value was 7.608. The p value came out to be statistically significant (p- 0.000). Pre test mean was 69.60 and post test mean was 66.00 for group C. The t value was 6.114. The p value was significant (p- 0.000). In Group D, pre test mean (M- 67.92) was slightly lower than post test mean (M- 68.40). The p-value was statistically non-significant (t- -0.690, p- 0.497).

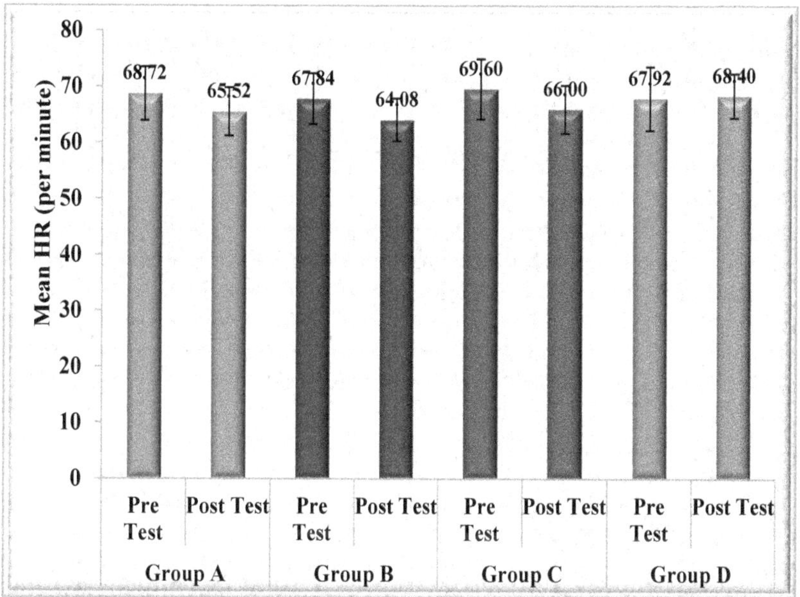

Figure 4.15: Pre and post test comparison for Heart rate

Mean and SD for the different groups in terms of heart rate is represented in Figure 4.15. In group A, pre test mean was 68.72 and post test mean was 65.52. SD for pre test was 4.79 and for post test was 4.33. In group B, mean in pre test was 67.84 and post test was 64.08. During pre test, SD was 4.50 and during post test, SD was 3.85. Mean in pre test was found to be 69.60 and in post test was 66.00 in group C. SD was 5.35 during pre test and 4.28 during post test. Mean during pre test was 67.92 and post test was 68.40 for Control group. SD was 5.67 during pre test and 3.95 during post test.

Table 4.43 : Descriptive Statistics of Groups without Adjusted Mean for Resting Heart Rate

Dependent Variable: Heart rate(per minute)			
Group	**N**	**Mean**	**Std. Deviation**
Group A	25	65.52	4.33
Group B	25	64.08	3.85
Group C	25	66.00	4.28
Group D	25	68.40	3.95
Total	100	66.00	4.33

The Table 4.43 depicts the descriptive statistics related to heart rate without adjusted covariate. During post-test mean heart rate of Group A was 65.52 ± 4.33, which was slightly less than Group C(66 ± 4.28). Resting Heart rate among students of Group D was maximum 68.40 ± 3.95 and minimum average was found in Group B (64.08 ± 3.85).

Table 4.44 : Equality of Error Variance among Groups in their Resting Heart Rate

Dependent Variable: Heart rate(per minute)			
F	**df1**	**df2**	**Sig.**
0.279	3	96	0.840^{NS}

NS- Non-Significant (p>0.05)

The Table 4.44 illustrates the equality of variance among the groups. The value of F is 0.279 which is not significant(p=0.840) at 0.05 level of Alpha. Test the null hypothesis that the error variance of the dependent variable is equal across groups. Therefore, the null hypothesis that there is an equal variance across groups is accepted.

Table 4.45 : Analysis of Covariance among Groups for Post Intervention Resting Heart Rate

Dependent Variable: Heart rate(per minute)						
Source	**Type III Sum of Squares**	**Df**	**Mean Square**	**F**	**Sig.**	**Partial Eta Squared**
Corrected Model	1374.044[a]	4	343.511	66.605	0.000	0.737
Intercept	209.054	1	209.054	40.535	0.000	0.299
HEART_RATE_PRE	1132.124	1	1132.124	219.513	0.000	0.698
GROUPS	272.035	3	90.678	17.582	0.000^{S}	0.357
Error	489.956	95	5.157			
Total	437464.000	100				
Corrected Total	1864.000	99				
a. R Squared = .737 (Adjusted R Squared = .726)						

S- Significant (p<0.05)

The table 4.45 reveals that the calculated value of F for group interaction was 17.582 which were statistically significant at 0.05 level of alpha. The F value illustrates significant difference in post intervention regarding Resting Heart Rate between the selected groups after adjusted the covariate pretest of respective variable. Therefore, the adjusted mean are significantly varies among the groups after covariate the pretest. The groups explained 73% variation for heart rate during post-test.

Table 4.46: Post Hoc Analysis of Heart rate(per minute)

(I) GROUPS	(J) GROUPS	Mean Difference (I-J)	Std. Error	p-value
Group A(Yoga Asana)	Group B	0.848	0.644	0.191^NS
	Group C	0.112	0.644	0.862^NS
	Group D	-3.419	0.643	0.000^S
Group B(Pranayama)	Group C	-0.735	0.647	0.259^NS
	Group D	-4.266	0.642	0.000^S
Group C(Asana and Pranayama Mixed Group)	Group D	-3.531	0.647	0.000^S

S- Significant($p<0.05$) NS- Non-Significant($p>0.05$)

Post hoc analysis of heart rate in Table 4.46 shows that all three training groups were having non-significant mean difference with each other. But students of Control group D were having significantly more heart rate than each training group

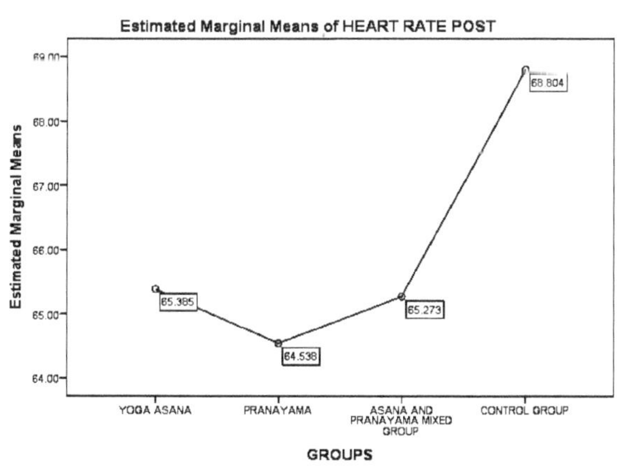

Figure 4.16 : Adjusted Mean Plot for resting heart rate during post-test

Mean plot in Figure 4.16, clearly shows that among all training groups, Pranayama helped a lot to improve the heart rate of students.

4. Breath holding capacity:

Breath holding capacity of students in seconds was evaluated during study.

Table 4.47 : Average breath holding capacity(seconds) among groups in pre-test

Group	N	Mean	Std. Deviation	Levene Statistic	p-value
Group A	25	49.57	9.26	0.937	0.426^{NS}
Group B	25	46.05	8.75		
Group C	25	43.51	6.94		
Group D	25	44.40	8.46		
Total	100	45.88	8.59		

NS- Non-Significant(p>0.05)

While analyzing breath holding capacity of students in Table 4.47 among various groups, It was noticed that mean was maximum in Group A(M-49.57) and minimum in Group C(M-43.51). In homogeneity test non-significant p-value(p=0.426; p>0.05) was calculated.

Table 4.48 : Pre and post comparison of breath holding capacity(seconds)

Group		N	Mean	SD	Mean difference	t	df	p-value
Group A	Pre Test	25	49.57	9.26	-3.130	-5.628	24	0.000^{S}
	Post Test	25	52.70	9.55				
Group B	Pre Test	25	46.05	8.75	-5.178	-7.869		0.000^{S}
	Post Test	25	51.23	9.92				
Group C	Pre Test	25	43.51	6.94	-4.386	-6.762		0.000^{S}
	Post Test	25	47.90	7.07				
Group D	Pre Test	25	44.40	8.46	-0.032	-0.056		0.956^{NS}
	Post Test	25	44.43	8.18				

S- Significant (p<0.05) NS- Non-Significant (p>0.05)

The table 4.48 shows the pre and post test comparison for breath holding capacity. In group A, pre test mean (M- 49.57) was lower than post test mean (M- 52.70).. The t value was -5.628. The p value came out to be significant (p-0.000). In group B, pre test mean was 46.05 and post test mean was 51.23. The mean difference and t value were -5.178 and -7.869 respectively. The p value was significant (p- 0.000). Pre test mean was 43.51 and post test mean was 47.90 for group C. The t value was -6.762. The p value was significant (p- 0.000). In control, pre test mean (M- 44.40) was lower than post test mean (M- 44.43). The mean difference and t value were -0.032 and -0.056 respectively. The p-value was statistically non-significant (p- 0.956 ; p>0.05).

Figure 4.17 represented change in mean breath holding capacity of students before and after intervention. In group A, pre test mean was 49.57 and post test mean was 52.70. In group B, mean in pre test was 46.05 and post test was 51.23. Mean in pre test was found to be 43.51 and in post test was 47.90 in group C. Mean during pre test was 44.40 and post test was 44.43 for Group D. Where breath holding capacity of training group improved significantly in post-test, little change was seen in control group.

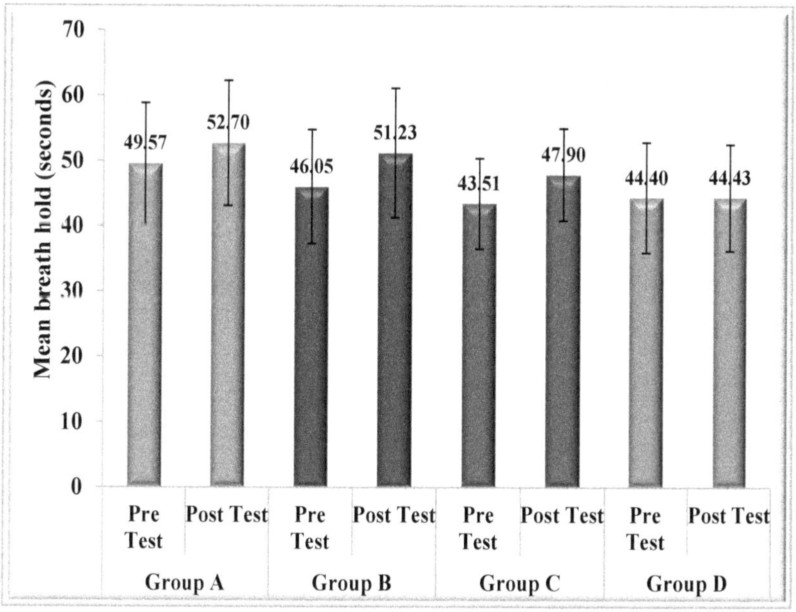

Figure 4.17: Pre and post test comparison for breath holding capacity

Table 4.49: Descriptive Statistics of Breath Holding Capacity without Adjusted Mean

Dependent Variable: Breath Holding Capacity(seconds)			
Group	**N**	**Mean**	**Std. Deviation**
Group A	25	52.70	9.55
Group B	25	51.23	9.92
Group C	25	47.90	7.07
Group D	25	44.43	8.18
Total	100	49.06	9.20

The Table 4.49 depicts the descriptive statistics in terms of mean and standard deviation without adjusted covariate. The mean and standard deviation during post-test of Group A was 52.70 ± 9.55, for Group B was 51.23 ± 9.92, for Group C was 47.90 ± 7.07 and mean and Standard Deviation of Group D was 44.43 ± 8.18 respectively. After intervention Group A students possessed maximum breath holding capacity, followed by Group B.

Table 4.50: Equality of Error Variance of Breath Holding among Groups

Dependent Variable: Breath Holding Capacity(seconds)			
F	**df1**	**df2**	**Sig.**
0.272	3	96	0.845^{NS}

NS- Non-Significant ($p>0.05$)

The Table 4.50 illustrates the equality of variance among the groups. The value of F is 0.272 which is not significant at 0.05 level of Alpha. Therefore, the null hypothesis that regarding equal variance across groups is accepted.

Table 4.51 : Analysis of Covariance among Groups for Post Intervention Breath Holding Capacity

Dependent Variable: Breath Holding Capacity(seconds)						
Source	**Type III Sum of Squares**	**Df**	**Mean Square**	**F**	**Sig.**	**Partial Eta Squared**
Corrected Model	7488.020[a]	4	1872.005	198.893	0.000	0.893
Intercept	55.502	1	55.502	5.897	0.017	0.058
BREATH_HOLD_PRE	6470.068	1	6470.068	687.418	0.000	0.879
GROUPS	385.946	3	128.649	13.668	0.000[S]	0.301
Error	894.153	95	9.412			
Total	249158.849	100				
Corrected Total	8382.173	99				
a. R Squared = .893 (Adjusted R Squared = .889)						

S- Significant (p<0.05)

In Table 4.51 it was observed that different interventions statistically considerable having adjusted for covariate. calculated value of F as 13.668 which were statistically significant at 0.05 level of alpha. The F value illustrate significant difference in post intervention of Breath Holding Capacity between the selected groups after adjusted the covariate pretest of respective variable. Therefore, the adjusted mean are significantly varies among the groups after covariate the pretest. The results revealed 89% strength for relationship of pre-test breath holding and group with post-intervention.

Table 4.52 : Post Hoc Analysis of Breath Holding Capacity(seconds)

(I) GROUPS	**(J) GROUPS**	**Mean Difference (I-J)**	**Std. Error**	**p-value**
Group A(Yoga Asana)	Group B	-1.969	0.878	0.027[S]
	Group C	-1.120	0.897	0.215[NS]
	Group D	3.215	0.889	0.000[S]
Group B(Pranayama)	Group C	0.849	0.873	0.333[NS]
	Group D	5.183	0.870	0.000[S]
Group C(Asana and Pranayama Mixed Group)	Group D	4.334	0.868	0.000[S]

S- Significant(p<0.05) NS- Non-Significant(p>0.05)

The table 4.52 shows the pair wise comparison of mean breath holding capacity among four groups. The mean difference of Group A (Yoga Asana) with Group B(Pranayama) was -1.969 and significant, but mean difference with Group C(mixed) was -1.120 which was not significant and mean difference with Group D(control group) was 3.215 which was significant at .05 level of alpha. Group B and Group C had non-significant mean difference (0.849). Group D was lagging behind all training groups significantly.

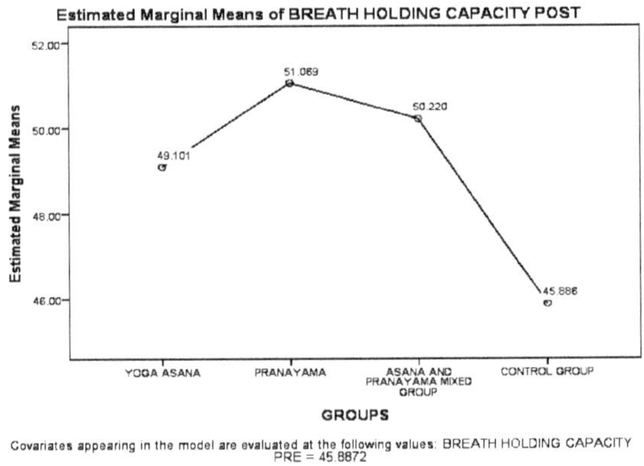

Figure 4.18 : Adjusted Mean Plot for Breath Holding Capacity

The Figure 4.18 highlighted that pranayama group shows higher mean difference with the control group.

SECTION – III ANALYSIS OF HEMATOLOGICAL VARIABLES

For, Objectives:

1. To ascertain the effects of yoga asana training, pranayama training and asana & pranayama combined training on haematological variables of their respective group.
2. To find out that which training has better effects on haematological variables within asana training, pranayama training and asana & pranayama combined training.

(Null Hypotheses):

1. There would be no significant difference in haematological variables on yoga asana group, pranayama group and asana & pranayama combined group due to their respective hatha yoga trainings.

2. It was hypothesized that asana training, pranayama training and asana & pranayama combined training equally effects the haematological variables of their respective group.

1. White blood cell

Hematological variable White blood cells was included in the study for evaluating health of students. Measuring unit for WBC was 10^3/uL.

Table 4.53 : Mean WBC(10^3/uL)among groups in pre-test

Group	N	Mean	Std. Deviation	Levene Statistic	p-value
Group A	25	6.90	1.27	0.607	0.612^{NS}
Group B	25	7.41	1.63		
Group C	25	7.07	1.49		
Group D	25	7.47	1.54		
Total	100	7.21	1.48		

NS- Non-Significant(p>0.05)

Table 4.53, shows that pre-test average White blood cell count among groups followed homogenous trend(p=0.612 ; p>0.05). Group A(M-6.90) having minimum and Group D(M-7.47) having maximum mean WBC were falling in same subset.

Table 4.54 : Pre and post comparison of WBC(10^3/uL)

Group	Test	N	Mean	SD	Mean difference	t	df	p-value
Group A	Pre Test	25	6.90	1.27	0.028	0.116	24	0.909^{NS}
	Post Test	25	6.88	1.43				
Group B	Pre Test	25	7.41	1.63	-0.036	-0.072		0.943^{NS}
	Post Test	25	7.44	2.09				
Group C	Pre Test	25	7.07	1.49	-0.332	-0.996		0.329^{NS}
	Post Test	25	7.40	1.60				
Group D	Pre Test	25	7.47	1.54	0.068	0.196		0.847^{NS}
	Post Test	25	7.40	2.24				

NS- Non-Significant (p>0.05)

The Table 4.54 shows the pre and post test comparison for WBC. In group A, pre test mean (M- 6.90) was slightly higher than post test mean (M-6.88). The mean difference and t value were 0.028 and 0.116 respectively. The p value came out to be non-significant (p- 0.909). In group B, students during pre test mean (M- 7.41) had the almost same white blood cells as students during post test (M- 7.44). The t value was -0.072. The p value came out to be non-significant (p- 0.943). Pre test mean WBC(M-7.07) increased to 7.40 in post test for group C but p value was non-significant (p- 0.329). In Group D, pre test mean (M- 7.47) reduced to 7.52 during post test. The mean difference and t value were -0.068 and 0.196 respectively. The p-value was statistically non-significant (p- 0.847).

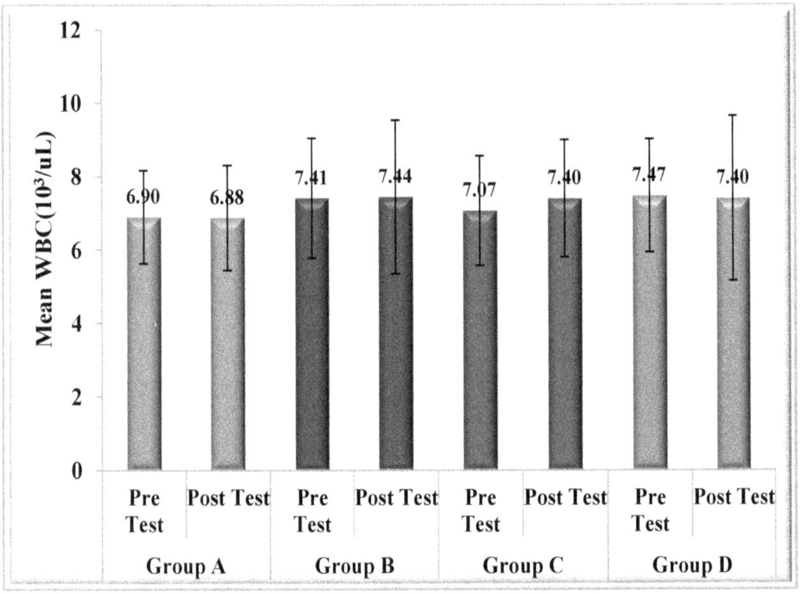

Figure 4.19: Pre and post test comparison for White Blood cells

Mean comparison of WBC in pre-test and post-test has been shown in Figure 4.19. In group A, pre test mean was 6.90 and post test mean was 6.88. In group B, WBC mean during both pre test and post-test was 7.41 and 7.44 respectively. Mean in pre test was found to be 7.07 and in post test was 7.40 in group C. Mean during pre test was 7.47 and post test was 7.40 for Control group. It was observed that Group B and Group C were able to mark some improvement in WBC whereas slight decrease in WBC was visible in Group A and D.

Table 4.55 : Descriptive Statistics of White Blood Cells without Adjusted Mean

Dependent Variable: White Blood Cells (cells/mcL)			
Group	**N**	**Mean**	**Std. Deviation**
Group A	25	6.88	1.43
Group B	25	7.44	2.09
Group C	25	7.40	1.60
Group D	25	7.40	2.24
Total	100	7.28	1.86

The Table 4.55 depicts the descriptive statistics in terms of mean and standard deviation without adjusted covariate. It was take into notice that mean and standard deviation of posttest of Group A was 6.88 ± 1.43, for Group B was 7.44 ± 2.09, for Group C was 7.40 ± 1.60 and mean and Standard Deviation of Group D was 7.40 ± 2.24 respectively. Among all 100 students average WBC was 7.28 ± 1.86.

Table 4.56 : Equality of Error Variance of White Blood Cells among Groups

Dependent Variable: WHITE BLOOD CELL Posttest			
F	**df1**	**df2**	**Sig.**
2.551	3	96	0.060[NS]

NS- Non-Significant (p>0.05)

The Table 4.56 illustrates the equality of variance among the groups. The value of F is 2.551 which is not significant at 0.05 level of Alpha. Therefore, the null hypothesis that there is an equal variance across groups is accepted.

Table 4.57 : Analysis of Covariance of White Blood Cells after Adjusted Mean among Groups

Dependent Variable: WHITE BLOOD CELL POST						
Source	**Type III Sum of Squares**	**Df**	**Mean Square**	**F**	**Sig.**	**Partial Eta Squared**
Corrected Model	66.292[a]	4	16.573	5.685	0.000	0.193
Intercept	46.422	1	46.422	15.925	0.000	0.144
WBC_PRE	60.771	1	60.771	20.848	0.000	0.180
GROUPS	2.508	3	0.836	0.287	0.835[NS]	0.009
Error	276.928	95	2.915			
Total	5651.800	100				
Corrected Total	343.220	99				
a. R Squared = .193 (Adjusted R Squared = .159)						

NS- Non-Significant (p>0.05)

The table 4.57 reveals that different interventions were statistically considerable having adjusted for covariate. It was observed that the calculated value of F for group's interaction was 0.287 which was not statistically significant at 0.05 level of alpha. The F value illustrates significant difference in post intervention of White Blood Cells between the selected groups after adjusted the covariate pretest of respective variable. Therefore, the adjusted mean are significantly varies among the groups after covariate the pretest.

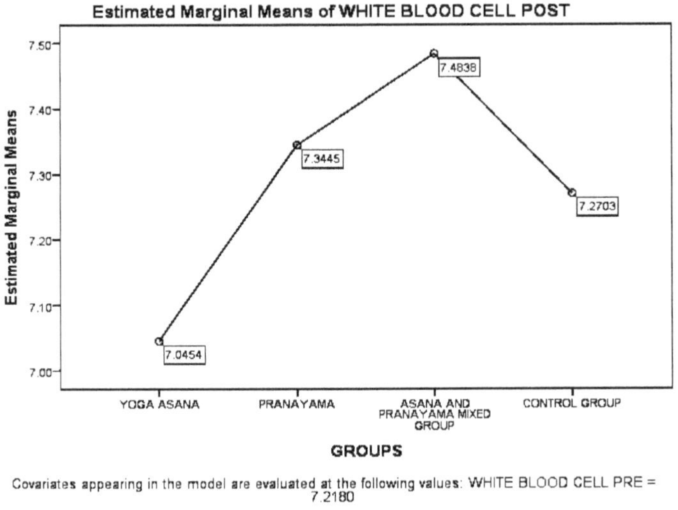

Figure 4.20 : Adjusted Mean Plot for White Blood Cells

The adjusted means for WBC among students in Figure 4.20 pointed out that Yoga asana and pranayama mixed training can help in increasing WBC.

2. Red Blood cell

Another hematological variable Red Blood cells, included in the study was measured in (10^6/uL).

Table 4.58 : Mean RBC(10^6/uL)among groups in pre-test

Group	N	Mean	Std. Deviation	Levene Statistic	p-value
Group A	25	4.41	0.57	1.930	0.130^{NS}
Group B	25	4.57	0.73		
Group C	25	4.49	0.39		
Group D	25	4.54	0.40		
Total	100	4.50	0.53		

NS- Non-Significant(p>0.05)

Pre intervention mean RBC count depicted in Table 4.58 were non-significantly(p=0.130; p>0.05) varying from each other. Maximum mean RBC were found in Group B(M-4.57), followed by Group D(M-4.54). Least mean RBC were noticed in Group A(M-4.41). The mean RBC for whole study population was 4.50 ± 0.53.

Table 4.59 : Pre and post comparison of RBC (10^6/uL)

Group		N	Mean	SD	Mean difference	t	df	p-value
Group A	Pre Test	25	4.41	0.57	-0.142	-0.994	24	0.330^{NS}
	Post Test	25	4.56	0.52				
Group B	Pre Test	25	4.57	0.73	0.036	0.260		0.797^{NS}
	Post Test	25	4.54	0.62				
Group C	Pre Test	25	4.49	0.39	-0.147	-2.136		0.043^{NS}
	Post Test	25	4.63	0.34				
Group D	Pre Test	25	4.54	0.40	-0.013	-0.171		0.866^{NS}
	Post Test	25	4.55	0.44				

NS- Non-Significant (p>0.05)

The Table 4.59 shows the pre and post test comparison for RBC. In group A, pre test mean was 4.41 and post test mean was 4.56. The mean difference and t value were -0.142 and -0.994 respectively. The p value came out to be non-significant (p- 0.330). In group B, pre test mean was 4.57 and post test mean was 4.54. The t value was

0.260. The p value came out to be statistically non-significant (p- 0.797). Pre test mean (M- 4.49) was less than post test mean (M- 4.63) for group C. The p value was significant (t- -2.136, p- 0.043). In control, pre test mean (M- 4.54) was slightly less than post test mean (M- 4.55). The mean difference and t value were -0.013 and -0.171 respectively. The p-value was statistically non-significant (p- 0.866).

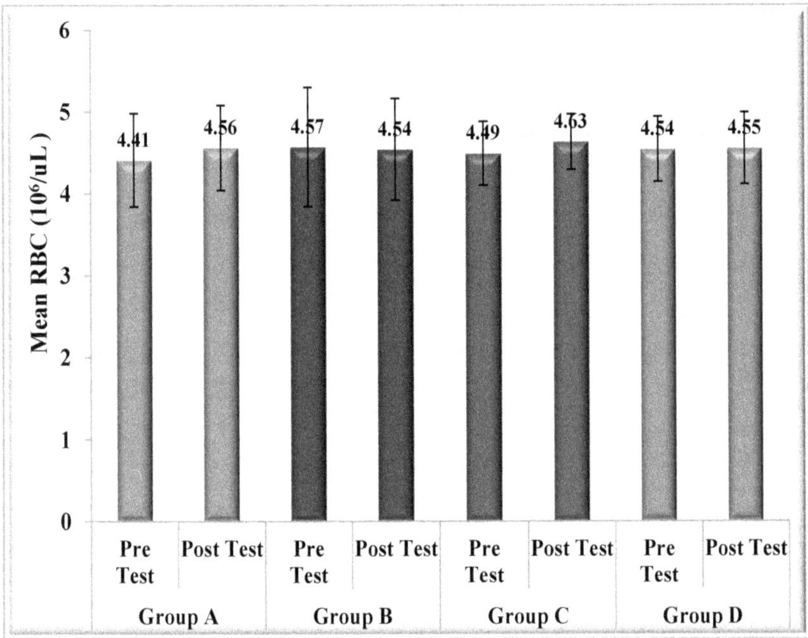

Figure 4.21: Pre and post test comparison for Red Blood cells

Mean and SD for the different groups in terms of RBC is represented in Figure 4.21. In group A, pre test mean was 4.41 and post test mean was 4.56. In group B, mean in pre test was 4.57 and post test was 4.54. Mean in pre test was found to be 4.49 and in post test was 4.63 in group C. Mean during pre test was 4.54 and post test was 4.55 for Control group. SD was 0.58 during pre test and 0.51during post test. Except Group B, all other groups showed increment in Red blood cells of students during post-test. Major change was noticed in Group C and Group A.

Table 4.60 : Descriptive Statistics of Red Blood Cells without Adjusted Mean

Dependent Variable: Red Blood Cells(10^6/uL)			
Group	**N**	**Mean**	**Std. Deviation**
Group A	25	4.56	0.52
Group B	25	4.54	0.62
Group C	25	4.63	0.34
Group D	25	4.55	0.44
Total	100	4.57	0.49

The Table 4.60 depicts the descriptive statistics in terms of mean and standard deviation without adjusted covariate. It was take into notice that mean and standard deviation of posttest of Group A was 4.56 ± 0.52, for Group B was 4.54 ± 0.62, for Group C was 4.63 ± 0.34 and mean and Standard Deviation of Group D was 4.55 ± 0.44 respectively. Mean RBC of 100 students was 4.57 ± 0.49

Table 4.61 : Equality of Error Variance of Red Blood Cells among Groups

Dependent Variable: Red Blood Cells(10^6/uL)			
F	**df1**	**df2**	**Sig.**
4.835	3	96	0.004^S

S- Significant ($p<0.05$)

The Table 4.61 illustrates the equality of variance among the groups. The value of F is 4.835 which is significant at 0.05 level of Alpha. Therefore, the null hypothesis that there is an equal variance across groups is rejected for RBC among students during post-test

The table 4.62 presents that different interventions were statistically considerable having adjusted for covariate. It was observed that the calculated value of F for group's interaction was 0.395 which was not statistically significant at 0.05 level of alpha. The F-value not illustrates significant difference in post intervention of Red Blood Cells between the selected groups after adjusted the covariate pretest of respective variable. Therefore, the adjusted means were not significantly varies among the groups after covariate the pre-test. Low 18% variation in post test RBC was explained by study groups.

Table 4.62 : Analysis of Covariance or Red Blood Cells after Adjusted the Mean

Dependent Variable: Red Blood Cells(10^6/uL)						
Source	Type III Sum of Squares	df	Mean Square	F	Sig.	Partial Eta Squared
Corrected Model	4.351[a]	4	1.088	5.298	0.001	0.182
Intercept	11.073	1	11.073	53.935	0.000	0.362
RBC_PRE	4.213	1	4.213	20.521	0.000	0.178
GROUPS	.243	3	0.081	0.395	0.757[NS]	0.012
Error	19.503	95	0.205			
Total	2117.008	100				
Corrected Total	23.854	99				
a. R Squared = .182 (Adjusted R Squared = .148)						

NS- Non-Significant (p>0.05)

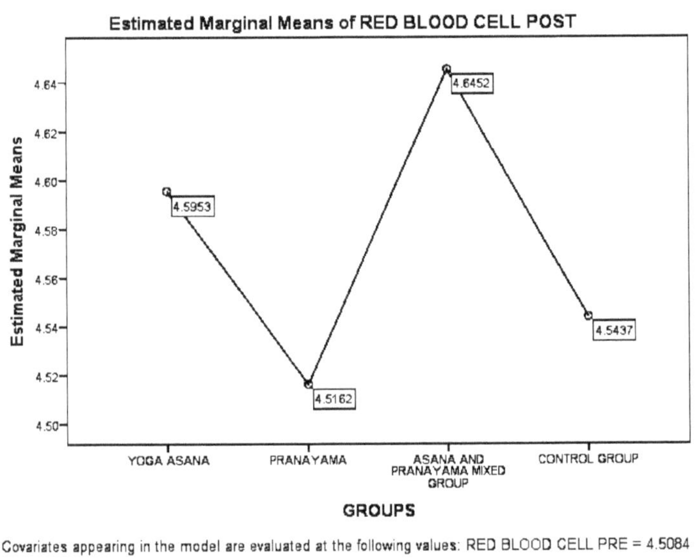

Figure 4.22 : Adjusted Mean Plot for Red Blood Cells of Different Groups

Figure 4.22 indicates that Yoga asana training is good but mixed yoga asana and pranayama training significant increase RBC among students.

3. Hemoglobin

Hemoglobin among students plays important role in their overall development. Therefore researcher had attempted to include Hemoglobin in study using g/dL unit.

Table 4.63 : Mean Hemoglobin(g/dL) among groups in pre-test

Group	N	Mean	Std. Deviation	Levene Statistic	p-value
Group A	25	11.22	1.52	1.554	0.206^{NS}
Group B	25	11.21	1.40		
Group C	25	11.27	1.05		
Group D	25	11.65	1.32		
Total	100	11.34	1.33		

NS- Non-Significant($p>0.05$)

The pre-test findings in Table 4.63 shows mean hemoglobin level of students in various groups. Maximum hemoglobin was observed in Group D (M-11.65). Rest all three groups had little difference regarding hemoglobin level. Homogenous level of hemoglobin resulted in non-significant p-value (0.206) in pre-test

Table 4.64 : Pre and post comparison of Hemoglobin (gm/dL)

Group		N	Mean	SD	Mean difference	t	df	p-value
Group A	**Pre Test**	25	11.22	1.52	-0.896	-2.740	24	0.011^{S}
	Post Test	25	12.12	1.03				
Group B	**Pre Test**	25	11.21	1.40	-0.848	-2.750		0.011^{S}
	Post Test	25	12.06	1.17				
Group C	**Pre Test**	25	11.27	1.05	-0.984	-6.086		0.000^{S}
	Post Test	25	12.26	1.11				
Group D	**Pre Test**	25	11.65	1.32	-0.486	-2.305		0.030^{S}
	Post Test	25	12.14	1.16				

S- Significant ($p<0.05$)

The Table 4.64 shows the pre and post test comparison for Hemoglobin. In group A, pre test mean (M- 11.22) was lower than post test mean (M-12.12). The mean difference and t value were -0.896 and -2.740 respectively. The p value came out to be significant (p- 0.011). In group B, mean Hemoglobin during pre test was 11.21

which increased in post test (M-12.06). The t value was -2.750. The p value came out to be significant (p- 0.011). Pre test mean was 11.27 and post test mean was 12.26 for group C. The highly significant p-value (p- 0.000) showed large improvement in hemoglobin level. In Group D, pre test mean (M- 11.65) was lower than post test mean (M- 12.14). The mean difference and t value were -0.486 and -2.305 respectively. The p-value was statistically significant (p- 0.030).

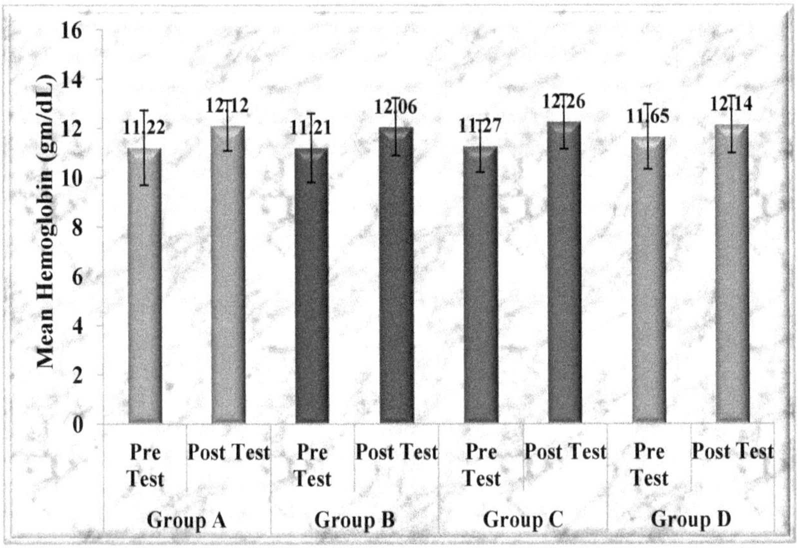

Figure 4.23: Pre and post test comparison for Hemoglobin

Mean difference in hemoglobin level of study groups during pre-test and post-test is presented through graph in Figure 4.23. In group A, pre test mean was 11.22 and post test mean was 12.12. In group B, mean in pre test was 11.21 and post test was 12.06. Mean in pre test was found to be 11.27 and in post test was 12.26 in group C. Mean during pre test was 11.65 and post test was 12.14 for Group D. It was concluded that students in all groups had significantly increased hemoglobin level during post-test compared to pre-test.

Table 4.65: Descriptive Statistics of Hemoglobin of Respondents of Different Groups

Dependent Variable: Hemoglobin (gm/dL)			
Group	**N**	**Mean**	**Std. Deviation**
Group A	25	12.12	1.03
Group B	25	12.06	1.17
Group C	25	12.26	1.11
Group D	25	12.14	1.16
Total	100	12.14	1.10

The Table 4.65 depicts the descriptive statistics in terms of hemoglobin among students without adjusted covariate. Mean hemoglobin during post-test of Group A was 12.12 ± 1.03, for Group B was 12.06 ±1.17, for Group C was 12.26 ± 1.11 and mean and Standard Deviation of Group D was 12.14± 1.16 respectively.

Table 4.66 : Equality of Error Variance of Hemoglobin among Groups

Dependent Variable: Hemoglobin (gm/dL)			
F	**df1**	**df2**	**Sig.**
0.484	3	96	0.694^{NS}

The Table 4.66 illustrates the equality of variance among the groups. The value of F is 0.484 which is not significant at 0.05 level of Alpha. Therefore, the null hypothesis for equal variance across groups is accepted.

Table 4.67 : Analysis of Covariance for Posttest of Hemoglobin with Covariate of Pretest among Different Groups

Dependent Variable: Hemoglobin(gm/dL)						
Source	**Type III Sum of Squares**	**Df**	**Mean Square**	**F**	**Sig.**	**Partial Eta Squared**
Corrected Model	24.958[a]	4	6.240	6.118	0.000	0.205
Intercept	81.695	1	81.695	80.099	0.000	0.457
HB_PRE	24.436	1	24.436	23.959	0.000	0.201
GROUPS	.893	3	0.298	0.292	0.831^{NS}	0.009
Error	96.892	95	1.020			
Total	14875.840	100				
Corrected Total	121.850	99				
a. R Squared = .205 (Adjusted R Squared = .171)						

NS- Non-significant (p>0.05)

The Table 4.67 reveals whether the different interventions were statistically considerable having adjusted for covariate. It was observed that the calculated value of F for group's interaction was 0.292 which was not statistically significant at 0.05 level of alpha. Therefore, the adjusted mean were not significantly varies among the groups after covariate the pretest. It was noticed that only 20% variation in hemoglobin was explained by groups.

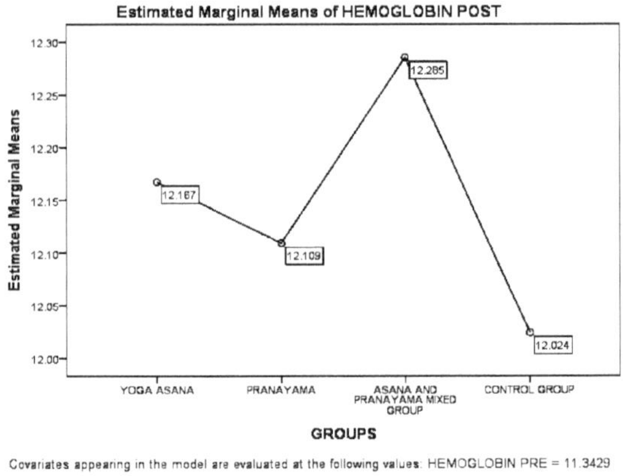

Figure 4.24 : Adjusted Mean Plot for Hemoglobin of Different Groups

Although all the study groups had mentioned increase in hemoglobin yet Group C(Yoga asana and pranayama mixed training) showed marked increase in hemoglobin of students more rapidly.

4. Platelets

Healthy platelet count ensures healthy life style. Here patelets were described in (10^3/uL).

Table 4.68 : Mean Platelets(10^3/uL) among groups in pre-test

Group	N	Mean	Std. Deviation	Levene Statistic	p-value
Group A	25	291.68	51.20	4.921	0.053^{NS}
Group B	25	290.16	66.27		
Group C	25	277.24	58.97		
Group D	25	303.36	93.54		
Total	100	290.61	69.26		

NS- Non-Significant(p>0.05)

Table 4.68 shows the platelets mean and standard deviation of various groups in pre-test. Group A had mean platelet count 291.68 and standard deviation 51.20 while Group had platelets 290.16±66.27. In group C, mean platelets and standard deviation was 277.24 and 58.97 respectively. Group D had mean platelets 303.36 and standard deviation 93.54. Total 100 students had mean 290.61 platelets. The p-value came out non-significant according to levene statistic (4.921).

Table 4.69 : Pre and post comparison of Platelets(10^3/uL)

Group		N	Mean	SD	Mean difference	T	df	p-value
Group A	Pre Test	25	291.68	51.20	10.880	1.317	24	0.200^{NS}
	Post Test	25	280.80	39.41				
Group B	Pre Test	25	290.16	66.27	13.640	0.990		0.332^{NS}
	Post Test	25	276.52	61.42				
Group C	Pre Test	25	277.24	58.97	-0.760	-0.074		0.942^{NS}
	Post Test	25	278.00	46.38				
Group D	Pre Test	25	309.36	93.54	24.160	1.843		0.078^{NS}
	Post Test	25	285.20	78.26				

NS- Non-Significant (p>0.05)

Pre and post test comparison for platelets is shown in the table 4.69. In group A, platelets mean was 291.68 during pre test and 280.80 during post test mean. The mean difference and t value were 10.880 and 1.317 respectively. The p value came out to be non-significant (p- 0.200). In group B, post test platelets mean (M- 290.16) was better than pre test platelets mean (M- 276.52). The t value was 0.990. The p value came out to be statistically non-significant (p- 0.332). Pre test mean was 277.24 and post test mean was 278.00 for group C. The t value was -0.074. The p value was non-significant (p- 0.942). In control group, pre test mean (M- 309.36) was slightly higher than post test mean (M- 285.20). The p-value was statistically non-significant (t-1.843, p- 0.078).

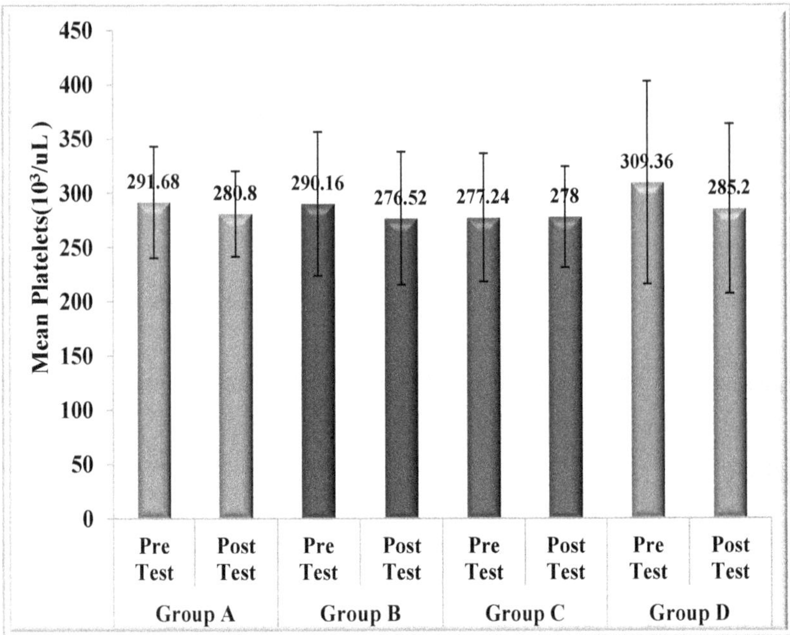

Figure 4.25: Pre and post test comparison for Hemoglobin

The above Figure 4.25 represent mean platelets count among various groups during pre and post-test. In group A, pre test mean was 291.68 and post test mean was 280.80. In group B, mean in pre test was 290.16 and post test was 276.52. Mean in pre test was found to be 277.24 and in post test was 278.00 in group C. Mean during pre test was 309.36 and post test was 285.20 for Control group. Platelets among Group A and B decreased during post-test. Little increase was noticed in Group C. But the decrease in Group D was little bigger among all groups.

Table 4.70: Descriptive Statistics of Platelets of Respondents at their Post Phase of Measurement without Adjusted Mean

Dependent Variable: Platelets(10^3/uL)			
Group	**N**	**Mean**	**Std. Deviation**
Group A	25	280.80	39.41
Group B	25	276.52	61.42
Group C	25	278.00	46.37
Group D	25	285.20	78.26
Total	100	280.13	57.52

The Table 4.70 depicts the descriptive statistics in terms of mean and standard deviation without adjusted covariate. Observations revealed that mean and standard deviation during post-test of Group A was 280.80 ± 39.41, for Group B was 276.52 ± 61.42, for Group C was 278 ± 46.37 and mean and Standard Deviation of Group D was 285.20 ± 78.26 respectively.

Table 4.71 : Equality of Error Variance of Platelets

Dependent Variable: Platelets(10^3/uL)			
F	**df1**	**df2**	**Sig.**
2.448	3	96	0.068[NS]

NS- Non-Significant (p>0.05)

The Table 4.71 illustrates the equality of variance among the groups. The value of F is 2.448 which is not significant at 0.05 level of Alpha. Therefore, the null hypothesis that there is an equal variance across groups is accepted.

The table 4.72 reveals whether the different interventions were statistically considerable having adjusted for covariate. It was observed that the calculated value of F for group's interaction was 0.186 which was not statistically significant at 0.05 level of alpha.

Table 4.72 : Analysis of Covariance for Platelets after Adjusting Mean

Dependent Variable: Platelets(10^3/uL)						
Source	**Type III Sum of Squares**	**df**	**Mean Square**	**F**	**Sig.**	**Partial Eta Squared**
Corrected Model	119121.889[a]	4	29780.472	13.572	0.000	0.364
Intercept	90096.470	1	90096.470	41.060	0.000	0.302
PLATLETS_PRE	118028.819	1	118028.819	53.789	0.000	0.362
GROUPS	1225.293	3	408.431	0.186	0.906[NS]	0.006
Error	208457.421	95	2194.289			
Total	8174861.000	100				
Corrected Total	327579.310	99				
a. R Squared = .364 (Adjusted R Squared = .337)						

NS- Non-Significant (p>0.05)

Therefore, the adjusted means were not significantly varies among the groups. The groups and pre-test platelet counts explained 36% variation in post-test mean platelet count results.

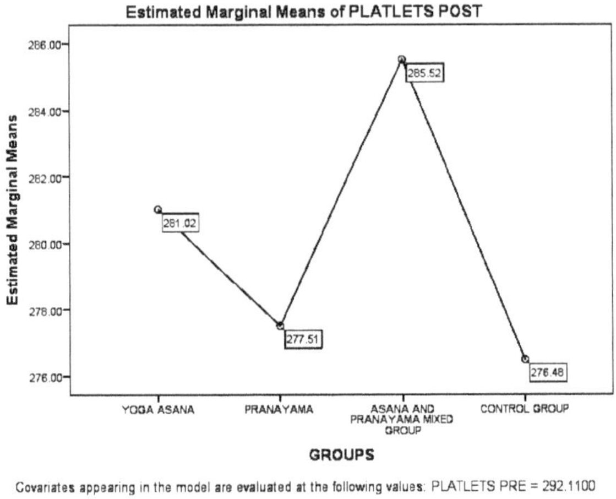

Figure 4.26 : Adjusted Mean Plot for Platelets

The mean plot of post-test platelet count proves Yoga asana and pranayama training better than other as this group maintained the platelet count level.

DISCUSSION ON FINDINGS

The purpose of the present study was to examine the Effect of Hatha Yoga on Physical Fitness, Physiological and Hematological Variables of School Level Students. To accomplish the study, a systematically procedure of experimental research was adopted. A total 100 sample were drawn out of population and quarterly divided into four groups. Each group was randomly formed consisting of 25 subjects in each group. Group A was assigned yoga Asana training, group B was subjected to Pranayama training and group C was provided Yoga Asana and Pranayama combination for the duration of 12 weeks with five days per week while group D was monitored as control group. The control group did not participate in any training programme. The analysis of covariance was used to find out the effects of different training on dependent variable. The following findings were observed as per the obtained results:

PHYSICAL FITNESS VARIABLES

In the aspect of speed (50 meter dash) a noticeable decrease was observed in the time of 50 meter dash after the training among the groups. After ensuring equal error variance among the groups it was observed during post-test that all three training programmes significantly improved the speed of students but control group improved non-significantly. The training groups were significantly better than control group for enhancing speed of students. Yoga asana and pranayama mixed training was found highly effective with minimum adjusted mean (M-7.71 seconds) time taken for 50 meter dash run.

The strength was measured through the standing broad jump. The significant enhancement of mean strength compared to pre-test was observed in all the three training groups except control group. Yoga Asana (Mean=1.92 m) group shows higher effect among all.

In Agility, high mean difference was observed for Mixed Group though Yoga and pranayama both significantly improved agility contrary to Control Group. It was revealed that for enhancing agility mix training is better method as per the obtained outcomes.

It is a general consideration that Yoga trainings improve the flexibility which was statistically significant proved for all training groups during study. Pre-post mean difference(-2.344) was found maximum for Yoga asana group The mean difference between Control and Yoga Asana Group was highest among all the groups. Even adjusted mean for Yoga asana group was maximum among all.

The post-intervention results indicated significant effect of various training programmes on endurance among students. Mixed training of Asana and Pranayama has maximum effect on endurance with the mean difference of -122.800 between pre and post-test.

It was observed that yoga trainings were found significant at the selected physical components.

Similar study **Rani & Malik (2017), Johnbosco (2018), Swamy & Patil (2016).** All mentioned studies reported significant effects of yoga training on the physical fitness variables. The findings of the studies supported the results of present study.

PHYSIOLOGICAL VARIABLES

In physiological variables it was observed that Systolic Blood pressure among students from all groups reduced after training but only pranayama and mixed training could significantly affect SBP. Calculated value of F for group's interaction was 1.871 which illustrating no significant difference in post intervention of systolic blood pressure between the selected groups. Combination of yoga and pranayama controlled the SBP among students more successfully.

Diastolic Blood Pressure among students in all groups reduced during post-test but in only Group B (Pranayama) it was reduced significantly. The F value does not illustrate significant difference in post intervention of Diastolic Blood Pressure between the selected groups after adjusted the covariate pretest of respective variable. Mixed training having least adjusted mean was appeared best for controlling DBP.

All training groups significantly influenced the heart rate of students but reverse findings were noticed in control group during post-test. Various groups were significantly different in terms of post-test adjusted means for heart rate. Pranayama was influencing most the heart rate of students. The present study result agrees with the results of **Divya et al. (2017), Goel et al. (2016), Sharma et al. (2013), Kaur et al. (2001).** All mentioned studies reported a significant decrease in the resting heart rate after employing the yogic exercises.

The effect of yoga training was visible on breath holding capacity with significant mean comparison of before and after intervention results. It was observed that the calculated value of F for group's interaction was **13.668** which were statistically significant at 0.05 level of alpha. Pranayama group was having maximum adjusted mean and proved finest among all. The findings of the study are in agreement with the results of **Vishnu (2017), Ramesh (2016), Makwana et al. (1988).** All mentioned studies found similar results on the breath holding after yoga trainings.

HEMATOLOGICAL VARIABLES

None of the study groups had shown significant change in post-test White Blood cells count. It was very noticeable phenomenon that only .09% of effects size (effect of training) was observed on white blood cells which are key terms of our immune system, Yoga asana and pranayama mixed training was found helpful for increasing

WBC among students. Same result was found by **Banerjee et al. (2019), Rayat & Paul (2018).**

After the interval of 12 weeks Red Blood cells were not significantly changed in all four groups but largest change was observed in mixed training group. Similar pattern was followed for Red Blood Cells, like WBC where 1.2 % of effects of training were observed on RBC. Same result was found by **(Chandrashekhar, 2012).**

Hemoglobin increased significantly among all study groups than pre-test. Yoga Asana and Pranayama mixed training more effectively improved the hemoglobin level of students. The findings of the study agree with the studies reported by **Geetanjali et al. (2014), Jothi (2014)**, and **Carranque et al. (2012)** who reported a significantly increase in the hemoglobin after employing the yogic exercise.

Impact of various yoga training was found non-significant on Platelet count of students. Platelet plays an important role in human body the main function of platelets was to maintain the homeostasis in the body. The magnitude of trainings effects for platelets was only 0.6% observed which was not significant. Yet yoga asana and pranayama mixed training proved helpful in increasing platelets. Same result was found by **(Chandrashekhar, 2012).**

It was a perceptible fact that blood chemistry has not effects of yoga asana and pranayama. Various factors can affect the blood chemistry or internal homeostasis such as diet, lifestyle, etc. maybe these cannot be controlled in the present study. It was recommended for the further studies that experimental studies need much focus on controlled environment.

TESTING OF HYPOTHESES

H_1: There would be no significant difference in physical fitness variables on yoga asana group, pranayama group and asana & pranayama combined group due to their respective hatha yoga trainings.

The study results showed significant effect of various trainings on speed of students. All training significantly enhanced the strength during study. Even the agility of students increased significantly in the training groups. Highly significant improvement in flexibility was observed as a result of different yoga trainings. Endurance among students increased significantly after 12 week yoga trainings.

The outcomes of the study shows that all the three experimental group shows significant positive effects on the selected physical fitness variables like speed, strength, agility, flexibility and endurance. So the hypothesis was rejected.

H_2: It was hypothesized that asana training, pranayama training and asana & pranayama combined training equally effects the physical fitness variables of their respective group.

While analyzing the study results it was seen that Yoga Asana and Pranayama mixed training was best for speed. Whereas Yoga asana proved best training for strength. Yoga asana and pranayama mixed training improved agility more effectively Yoga asana was the best training for flexibility. Mixed training was adjusted best for endurance.

It can be concluded from the study results that different training programmes were suitable for various physical fitness parameters. Thus the current hypothesis regarding equally effectiveness of trainings was rejected.

H_3: There would be no significant difference in physiological variables on yoga asana group, pranayama group and asana & pranayama combined group due to their respective hatha yoga trainings.

Among all training groups, pranayama and yoga asana and pranayama mixed training significantly controlled systolic blood pressure of students. Only significant impact of pranayama training was visible on Diastolic Blood Pressure. Various training programmes significantly decreased the heart rate of students. Breath holding capacity of students improved with all yoga trainings significantly.

In physiological variables all the three training groups succeeded to show significant effect differently. Yoga asana training failed to impact systolic and diastolic blood pressure significantly. But all trainings had significantly improved resting heart rate and breath holding capacity of students. Hence the hypothesis was partially rejected.

H_4: It was hypothesized that asana training, pranayama training and asana & pranayama combined training equally effects the physiological variables of their respective group.

Yoga asana and pranayama mixed training more successfully controlled Systolic blood pressure and Diastolic Blood Pressure. Whereas Pranayama effected more positively resting heart rate and breathing holding capacity.

The impact of different trainings in the study was not similar for all physiological variables SBP, DBP, Heart rate and breath holding capacity. Only Pranayama was effective for all parameters thus rejects the null hypothesis partially.

H_5 :. There would be no significant difference in haematological variables on yoga asana group, pranayama group and asana & pranayama combined group due to their respective hatha yoga trainings.

None of the training programme could significantly affect While Blood Cells and Red Blood Cells among students. Whereas Hemoglobin was significantly improved in all training groups. Even Platelet count of students was non-significantly changed with respective training programmes.

The outcomes of the study showed that all three types of trainings failed to show significant effects on all haematological variables except hemoglobin. All three trainings were similarly failed for most of the variables i.e WBC, RBC and platelets. So the null hypothesis was accepted partially.

H_6: It was hypothesized that asana training, pranayama training and asana & pranayama combined training equally effects the haematological variables of their respective group

Individual Yoga asana and Pranayama training failed to affect all hematological variables positively. Hemoglobin was significantly improved in all groups. All hematological variables White Blood Cells, Red Blood Cells, Hemoglobin and platelets were majorly increased with Yoga asana and pranayama mixed training. But difference between all three training groups was non significant

It was hypothesized that the entire three experimental groups showed similar effects on the selected haematological variables like white blood cell, red blood cell, hemoglobin and platelets. The outcomes of the study showed that all three types of trainings failed to show significant variance among groups on all haematological variables. So the null hypothesis was accepted.

SUMMARY OF THE CHAPTER:

In this chapter analysis of the data, interpretations of results and discussion on results have been presented. This chapter showed the effects of asana training, Pranayama training and asana & Pranayama combined training on physical fitness, physiological and haematological variables of students. It also showed which training has better effects or results on selected variables. In the next chapter summary of the study, findings and conclusions of the study were presented.

CHAPTER–V

SUMMARY, FINDINGS, CONCLUSIONS AND RECOMMENDATIONS

SUMMARY

Yoga is mixture of spiritual, mental and physical practice or tradition which originates in ancient India. Yogic practice has an excellent effect on physical and physiological parameters as per the previous research shown. A lot of space for the research is available in the field of Yoga with different parameters.

In the Present study four groups were randomly formed. Each group consists of 25 participants. The first group take part in Yoga Asana training, second groups was taking Pranayama training, third groups was performing mixture of yoga asana and pranayama training while the fourth groups act as control groups who did not take part in any training. Pretest and posttest was taken before and after the training provided of all groups including control group. To find out the best training method in comparison of control group analysis of co-variance was used as a part of general liner modal. The pretest was act as covariate for the present study. Physical, Physiological and Hematological variables were selected as dependent variables of the study while, the different training schedules were considered as independent variable for the present study.

The findings of the current study shows that various yoga trainings were significantly effective on physical fitness components like speed, strength, flexibility, endurance and agility and positively significant on physiological parameters like resting heart rate and breath holding capacity but not significant effect on blood pressure and except hemoglobin all hematological variables of the subjects.

FINDINGS

Following findings were observed after analysis the meaningful outcomes on the basis of attained data after the training provided.

FINDINGS IN PHYSICAL COMPONENTS

1. The pre-test and post-test mean comparison of speed produced highly significant results for Group A (Yoga Asana), Group B (Pranayama) and Group C (Yoga Asana and Pranayama mixed) training groups. But pre and post intervention mean comparison of Group D was non-significant (p-0.100) for speed. It was seen that all three trainings significantly improved the speed of students.
2. It was observed that the calculated value of F for group's interaction was 17.309 which were statistically significant at 0.05 level of alpha. The adjusted mean significantly varied among the groups after covariate the pretest. Maximum mean difference (0.502) was observed for Group C while paired sample t-test. and even the adjusted mean for post-test was minimum (M-7.71 seconds) for Group C compared to other groups indicating Yoga Asana and Pranayama mixed training best for speed.
3. Strength among students increased after three yoga trainings highly significantly. But non-significant improvement was noticed in control group.
4. The F value 31.775 for group's interaction illustrates significant difference in post intervention of Standing Broad Jump between the selected groups significant variation among the groups after covariate the pretest. With maximum adjusted mean (1.92m) Yoga asana proved best training for strength.
5. While assessing agility the mean time for training groups was significantly lower than pre-test contrarily in control group it non-significantly increased during post-test.
6. The adjusted mean were significantly different among the groups after covariate the pretest. In Group C maximum mean decrease was observed also adjusted mean was lowest with Yoga asana and pranayama mixed training proving it best for agility.
7. Flexibility of students increased during post-test but except control group(p-0.195) for all groups highly significant(p-0,000) p-value was calculated.
8. For Flexibility calculated value of F for group's interaction was 41.298 which were statistically significant. Yoga asana was found most impactful among all for flexibility with maximum adjusted mean 9.57.

9. It was observed during post-test that endurance among all training groups enhanced significantly but decline was seen in Control group.
10. The F value illustrates significant difference in endurance during post intervention of 12 Minute Run and Walk between the selected groups. Adjusted mean for mixed training was maximum (M-1968.7) showing it best among all for endurance.

FINDINGS IN PHYSIOLOGICAL VARIABLES

1. After 12 week training all study groups were showing decreased Systolic Blood pressure. It was seen that SBP decreased significantly with training in Group B (pranayama) and Group C(mixed).
2. It was observed that the calculated value of F for group's interaction was 1.871 which was not statistically significant at 0.05 level of alpha. Yoga asana and pranayama mixed training succeeded in controlling SBP more significantly with mean difference 1.400 and adjusted mean 117.39.
3. The effect of training on Diastolic Blood Pressure was visible in all the groups but significant impact was seen in Group B(Pranayama). The mean difference before and after intervention was maximum(1.520) for Group C(Yoga asana and pranayama).
4. It was observed that adjusted mean did not significantly varied among the groups after covariate the pretest. Rather maximum effect was seen with least adjusted mean (M-75.96) in Group C(Yoga asana and pranayama).
5. Significant decline in Heart rate of training groups was noticed during post-test but it increased for Group D(Control group). Group B(Pranayama) more efficiently improved heart rate of students with mean difference 3.760.
6. The adjusted mean significantly varied among the groups after covariate the pretest. Group B(Pranayama) having minimum adjusted mean(M-64.53) was more suitable training for heart rate.
7. Breath holding capacity of students improved with all training significantly but non-significantly in control group. Group B(Pranayama) had improved the breath holding of capacity of students most with 5.178 mean difference.

8. Significant difference in post intervention of Breath Holding Capacity between the selected groups after adjusted the covariate pretest of respective variable was observed. Highest adjusted mean (M-51.06) in Group B displayed the crucial role of Pranayama for improving breath holding capacity.

FINDINGS IN HEMATOLOGICAL VARIABLE

1. From the observations non-significant changes in White Blood Cells were noticed for all three training groups as well as control group. Where students in Group B and Group C had increased mean WBC, Group A had slight decline but Group D (Control) had larger decline in WBC.
2. It was observed that the calculated value of F for group's interaction was 0.287 indicating not significant variation among the groups. Largest increase in Group C (M-7.48) indicates that Yoga asana and pranayama mixed training is perfect for increasing WBC.
3. Except Group B, with non-significant but decreased, all other groups had non-significantly increased level of Red Blood Cells in post-test. Larger increase was noticed in mixed training group.
4. The F value 0.395 illustrates not significant difference in post intervention of Red Blood Cells between the selected groups after adjusted the covariate pretest of respective variable. With highest adjusted mean (M-4.64) yoga asana and pranayama mixed was found appropriate training for increased RBC.
5. Mean comparison between pre and post-test revealed significant difference in all groups for Hemoglobin. The great impact on hemoglobin was seen with yoga asana and pranayama mixed training having 0.984 highly significant mean difference.
6. Adjusted mean were not significantly varying among the groups after covariate the pretest. Group C (mixed training) was having highest adjusted mean(M-12.28) showing it more helpful for hemoglobin.
7. The results of the study revealed non-significant changes in Platelet count of students during pre-test and post-test. Maximum mean difference 13.640 was observed in Group B(Pranayama)

8. It was observed that the calculated value of F 0.186 illustrated non-significant difference in post intervention of Platelets between the selected groups after adjusted the covariate pretest of respective variable. Adjusted mean (M-285.62) was maximum resulted from yoga asana and pranayama mixed training.

The following findings given above were based on the outcomes of tables of between subjects factor which show the significant variation between different groups involved in the study. The brief description was given in the conclusions of the study the next main heading of this chapter.

CONCLUSIONS OF THE STUDY

The conclusion is proposed to help the reader comprehend why your research should matter to them afterward they have completed reading the thesis. A conclusion is not just a summary of your points or a re-statement of your research problem but a synthesis of key points.

1. It was concluded on the basis of the obtained outcomes that significance influence of Hath Yoga training on physical fitness variable was noticed after adjusted the mean values (covariate) therefore, the null hypothesis which was formulated earlier that "there is no significant difference in physical fitness variables on yoga asana group, pranayama group and asana pranayama combined group due to their respective hath yoga training with relatively control group" was not accepted. In Physical variables, Yoga asana was good for strength and flexibility but combined training of yoga asana and pranayama had effectively improved speed, agility and endurance among students.

2. In physiological variables the null hypothesis is falling to reject on some parameters for instance, diastolic and systolic blood pressure where training has similar effects. Whereas, resting heart rate and breath holding capacity has significant variation noticed after the given training. The Systolic blood pressure and Diastolic Blood Pressure showed positive impact of Yoga asana and pranayama mixed training but Pranayama was found most effective for heart rate and breath holding capacity.

3. In hematological variables all training groups have observed equal variance therefore, here; the researcher was failing to rejects the null hypothesis in each variable. Only hemoglobin increased significantly among all training groups after 12 weeks. Yoga asana and pranayama mixed training was found effective on all hematological variables like White Blood Cells, Red Blood Cells, Hemoglobin and platelets. Hematological parameters could be effected by various factors such as diet, rest, environment etc. which cannot be controlled properly during the training period. So, it may effects the results of the study that's why these factors should be considered as limitations of the study or beyond the control of the researcher.

RECOMMENDATIONS

Every research work has established some aim and objectives as per the nature of the study. The obtained consequences should bring meaningful and valuable phenomenon for the concerned population and society. These conclusions are important for our policy maker, social thinkers, govt. machineries who are responsible for betterment of sports environment in the nation. In the present study the following educational implications were suggested by the researcher on the basis of obtained consequences:

1. The yogic training should be implemented on the root level of the society for instance, in middle school to college or university level. Because these institutes are deals with the youth and healthy youth is the spine of every nation.

2. Yoga and physical education should be included in the curriculum of the each institute whether it should belong to engineering, science, medical science and art also.

3. The govt. authority should implement the means of yoga in each discipline of work to make the people healthy and fit and psychological wellbeing.

4. It is recommended that physical education teachers, trainers and coaches should give due importance to yoga and make it a part of their professional commitment.

5. New studies can be carried out to know the various effects of different yogic exercises combination.

6. Yoga, a form of mind- body work out, has become an increasingly well-known therapy used to maintain wellness, and alleviate a series of health problems and ailments. Yoga should be considered as a complementary treatment or alternative method for medical therapy in the treatment of different diseases.
7. Yoga suspends the fluctuations of the mind and by acting consciously, we live better and suffer less
8. Similar researcher can be conducted with different variables.
9. The experimental study should be more controlled in nature and scientific approach should as assessed.
10. The study should be conducted on different hematological parameters with different training plans.
11. Biomechanical analysis of Yogic movement can also be done
12. The present study was limited to male students only thus gender difference can be concluded only if females' students would be added.

APPENDIX-I

GROUP-A

(YOG ASANA)

PHYSICAL FITNESS VARIABLES

Subjects	50mts.dash run (Seconds)		Broad jump (Mts.)		Shuttle run (seconds)		Sit and reach (cm.)		12 minutes walk/run	
	PRE	POST	PRE	POST	PRE	POST	PRE	POST	PRE	POST
1	7.81	7.33	1.9	2.05	11.62	11.45	4.2	6.3	1960	2020
2	7.19	7.02	2.05	2.12	10.57	10.31	8.4	9.6	2240	2300
3	7.33	6.91	1.82	1.99	11.1	10.15	5.6	8.1	2320	2380
4	8.68	8.14	1.64	1.85	11.89	11.56	4	5.3	1960	2040
5	8.92	8.09	1.72	1.83	10.92	10.65	6.8	9.4	1980	2000
6	9.24	8.65	1.45	1.52	13.24	12.09	3.1	4	1860	1920
7	7.66	7.12	1.92	2.07	11.03	10.57	-2	1.6	1960	2060
8	8.21	8.04	1.43	1.67	11.68	10.65	4.1	8.9	2000	2120
9	7.36	7.13	1.56	1.78	11.4	10.28	7.5	8.9	1660	1720
10	8.15	7.52	1.75	1.95	12.16	11.52	10.3	12.9	1840	1800
11	8.61	8.11	1.42	1.57	12.24	11.02	13	15.2	1680	1740
12	9.85	9.21	1.36	1.68	11.81	10.43	3.7	8.6	1560	1680
13	8.38	8.26	1.51	1.75	11.38	10.12	4.1	7.5	1660	1720
14	8.82	8.17	1.67	1.78	11.74	11.29	6.3	8.4	1580	1640
15	9.32	8.97	1.62	1.76	12.15	11.17	5	7.3	1540	1680
16	8.45	8.1	1.98	2.14	11.96	11.02	14.9	15.2	1580	1640
17	7.42	7.14	1.65	1.87	12.08	12.15	7.9	9.1	1840	1960
18	7.12	7.15	1.91	1.98	11.47	11.25	11.5	13.4	1640	1720
19	8.1	7.28	1.6	1.75	12.2	10.91	2.9	6.8	1780	1900
20	8.05	7.83	1.65	1.73	12.07	12.12	9.7	12.5	1660	1700
21	8.09	7.65	1.75	1.94	11.67	11.28	10.5	12.7	1620	1720
22	7.45	6.83	1.62	1.78	11.36	10.42	8.2	9.6	2220	2380
23	8.1	7.38	1.71	1.86	12.3	11.58	16.8	20.1	2180	2240
24	7.13	6.02	1.95	2.1	10.97	10.34	10.2	13.5	2060	2200
25	7.75	7.28	2.1	2.15	10.91	10.86	8.6	9	1940	1960

GROUP-B

(PRANAYAMA GROUP)

PHYSICAL FITNESS VARIABLES

Subjects	50mts dash run (Seconds)		Broad jump (Mts.)		Shuttle run (seconds)		Sit and reach (Cm.)		12 minutes run/walk (Mts.)	
	PRE	POST	PRE	POST	PRE	POST	PRE	POST	PRE	POST
1	7.64	7.78	1.85	1.89	11.37	10.92	7.3	8.4	1940	2020
2	7.52	7.16	1.96	1.92	11.8	11.19	9.2	9.7	2240	2260
3	7.54	7.35	1.9	1.95	11.89	11.45	12.4	14.2	2320	2400
4	7.46	7.41	2.14	2.16	10.9	10.23	11.7	12.4	1980	2060
5	7.21	7.06	1.97	1.95	10.3	10.42	9.5	10.4	1980	1980
6	7.89	7.16	1.65	1.72	11.64	11.23	5.3	5.8	1860	1900
7	8.32	8.11	1.72	1.86	11.22	11.04	6.9	7.2	1960	2040
8	7.08	6.58	1.84	1.8	11.67	11.49	8.2	9.7	2000	2080
9	8.81	8.14	1.82	1.95	11.13	10.94	3.4	5.1	1660	1700
10	9.41	9.12	1.52	1.59	12.35	11.26	10.7	12.5	1840	1860
11	8.51	8.26	1.6	1.64	11.34	11.09	3.8	4.2	1680	1660
12	11.21	10.98	1.34	1.39	14.3	13.12	8.2	9.8	1520	1580
13	11.76	11.14	1.7	1.76	12.83	11.59	6.4	9	1660	1720
14	8.67	8.23	1.95	2	12.67	11.88	9.6	9.9	1580	1660
15	9.88	9.54	1.92	1.98	12.08	11.76	10.1	10.5	1540	1580
16	8.4	8.22	1.8	1.76	12.62	11.18	5.4	5.8	1560	1620
17	8.93	8.19	1.42	1.48	12.44	11.23	2.6	3.1	1840	1860
18	8.89	8.63	1.65	1.79	11.48	11.02	4.9	6.1	1640	1680
19	8.14	7.97	1.72	1.8	11.91	11.12	6.3	7.8	1780	1760
20	8.43	8.19	1.76	1.87	12.09	11.29	4.1	5.7	1660	1660
21	7.65	7.62	1.8	1.96	11.72	11.17	11.5	13.6	1640	1680
22	7.8	7.16	1.92	2.05	12.07	11.19	10.4	11.5	2220	2320
23	7.92	**7.56**	1.81	**1.94**	10.87	10.14	15.8	16.9	2180	2220
24	8.12	**8.04**	1.87	**1.99**	11.19	9.63	8.4	9.8	2060	2080
25	7.98	**7.56**	1.79	**1.86**	10.85	10.13	9.1	11.5	1940	2000

GROUP-C

(ASANA &PRANAYAMA MIX GROUP)

PHYSICAL FITNESS VARIABLES

Subjects	50mts dash run (Seconds)		Broad jump (Mts.)		Shuttle run (second)		Sit and reach (cm.)		12minutes run/walk (Mts.)	
	PRE	POST	PRE	POST	PRE	POST	PRE	POST	PRE	POST
1	**8.42**	8.21	2.02	2.19	10.01	9.24	11.2	13.5	2240	2340
2	**7.46**	7.49	2.12	2.26	9.81	9.04	12.3	14.1	1960	2020
3	**7.7**	7.1	1.98	2.06	10.9	10.86	14.5	15.4	2180	2260
4	**8.64**	8.42	1.68	1.86	11.83	10.21	-1.6	2.1	1860	1920
5	**6.61**	6.34	2.08	2.15	10.66	10.36	2.7	4.9	2320	2400
6	**8.49**	8.04	1.73	1.85	11.54	11.38	9.4	10.5	1760	1920
7	**7.46**	7.06	1.86	1.92	10.65	10.39	10.6	12	1680	1740
8	**8.83**	8.11	1.67	1.75	10.88	10.12	6.4	8.6	1840	1920
9	**7.92**	7.09	1.86	1.97	11.4	10.43	8.7	9.8	1980	2040
10	**8.5**	8.14	1.5	1.63	11.14	10.86	5.3	7	1760	1860
11	**8.44**	7.93	1.92	2.08	10.77	9.16	3.7	5	1780	1860
12	**8.83**	8.11	1.45	1.53	11.9	10.23	8.2	11	1860	1920
13	**8.8**	7.59	1.36	1.36	11.48	11.28	7.1	9.6	1740	1860
14	**8.12**	8.01	1.8	1.95	12.2	10.97	5	8.2	1860	2020
15	**7.22**	6.99	1.96	2.06	11.4	10.49	16.4	17.6	2320	2480
16	**7.74**	7.23	1.87	1.92	10.9	10.63	4.2	6.4	2060	2240
17	**8.52**	**7.85**	1.85	1.93	11.24	10.65	12.8	14.7	1840	1980
18	**8.8**	8.24	1.6	1.72	12.65	12.09	6.7	8.2	2280	2420
19	**8.17**	7.68	1.52	1.64	10.58	10.26	9.4	11.8	2020	2180
20	**8.73**	8.49	1.69	1.86	12.48	11.07	5.3	7.2	1960	2040
21	**7.96**	7.1	1.74	1.76	11.53	11.29	7.4	9.5	2000	2080
22	**7.44**	6.86	1.91	1.94	11.47	11.04	6.8	7.9	2160	2380
23	**7.7**	7.25	2.07	2.1	10.97	10.68	6.7	9.2	1880	1860
24	**8.42**	8.06	2.27	2.37	11.3	10.43	5.2	7.4	1920	2000
25	**8.23**	7.19	1.72	1.79	11.92	11.87	4.7	6.9	2180	2240

GROUP-D

(CONTROL GROUP)

PHYSICAL FITNESS VARIABLES

Sr No	50mts dash run (second)		Broad jump (mts.)		Shuttle run (second)		Sit and reach (c.m.)		12minutes run/walk (Mts.)	
	PRE	POST	PRE	POST	PRE	POST	PRE	POST	PRE	POST
1	7.41	7.28	1.94	1.9	11.46	11.52	7.2	7.4	1980	1920
2	7.92	7.88	1.9	1.96	12.06	12.02	5	5.2	1760	1780
3	8.13	8.28	1.75	1.74	12.42	12.46	4.3	4.1	1940	1960
4	6.25	6.17	2.43	2.4	10.23	10.04	18	17.8	2320	2260
5	7.18	7.2	2.05	2.15	11.49	11.65	9.2	9.1	1920	1940
6	8.1	7.96	1.78	1.75	12.13	12.05	5.5	5.8	1780	1720
7	8.42	8.46	1.92	1.95	12.21	12.18	-1	1	1660	1680
8	7.74	7.79	1.87	1.85	12.08	11.96	4.2	4.3	1780	1820
9	7.98	8.05	1.91	1.94	12.23	12.35	6.7	6.6	1600	1660
10	8.04	7.58	1.83	1.88	12.13	12.18	5.3	5.5	1720	1680
11	8.67	9.01	1.56	1.54	12.61	12.45	7.4	7.6	1680	1720
12	7.94	7.82	1.74	1.73	10.68	10.49	-1	0	1720	1660
13	8.23	8.28	1.96	1.98	11.59	11.85	3.8	3.5	1820	1880
14	9.88	9.45	1.34	1.4	13.27	13.16	9.5	9	1680	1660
15	9.71	9.68	1.5	1.53	12.88	12.67	4.8	4.6	1700	1760
16	8.21	8.14	1.72	1.69	12.53	12.69	4.2	4.1	1680	1660
17	7,9	7.54	1.82	1.84	12.18	12.06	7.8	7.8	1820	1860
18	8.48	8.36	1.93	1.9	12.14	12.23	5.2	5.8	1720	1660
19	7.62	7.58	1.9	1.95	11.4	11.17	8.7	8.9	1900	1860
20	8.55	8.64	1.65	1.61	11.52	11.26	4.1	4	1780	1820
21	8.74	8.82	1.55	1.56	12.98	12.62	8	8.1	1920	1860
22	7.63	7.39	1.72	1.7	11.26	11.23	3.8	3.5	2040	2020
23	8.22	8.19	1.98	2.02	12.07	12.26	2.7	2.4	1640	1600
24	9	9.15	1.45	1.43	12.2	12.06	5.2	5.8	1520	1560
25	8.48	8.06	1.68	1.71	12.47	12.29	7.4	7.5	1680	1660

GROUP-A

ASANA GROUP

PHYSIOLOGICAL VARIABLES

Subject	Systolic blood pressure/mmhg		Diastolic blood pressure/mmhg		Heart beat per/min.		breath holding cap. (sec.)	
	PRE	POST	PRE	POST	PRE	POST	PRE	POST
1	118	119	76	78	68	64	47.76	52.46
2	116	114	73	74	64	60	37.07	43.65
3	121	118	78	74	76	74	65.14	68.84
4	119	120	80	78	68	64	45.69	46.87
5	116	118	76	75	70	66	52.41	54.58
6	115	114	77	78	64	62	35.14	39.45
7	120	119	82	79	72	68	50.72	52.36
8	114	116	75	79	68	64	66.12	67.71
9	118	116	77	78	70	66	48.19	54.87
10	114	118	76	74	70	66	56.73	61.27
11	122	118	83	81	76	72	41.96	46.98
12	117	115	76	75	66	66	63.73	67.15
13	121	120	80	78	74	72	46.33	49.54
14	119	117	77	76	78	70	49.43	53.96
15	117	118	74	75	66	64	37.78	42.58
16	123	121	81	79	70	72	53.44	57.65
17	113	116	72	74	62	60	44.91	46.48
18	116	114	76	75	60	58	39.17	35.14
19	120	119	83	80	76	72	63.79	62.54
20	112	116	73	78	64	62	43.49	49.25
21	123	120	84	81	70	64	37.68	38.21
22	117	118	78	76	62	62	49.26	51.58
23	119	121	81	80	70	64	52.14	50.24
24	113	116	72	74	68	62	62.09	69.27
25	118	114	74	76	66	64	49.1	54.89

GROUP-B

(PRANAYAMA GROUP)

PHYSIOLOGICAL VARIABLES

Subjects	Systolic blood pressure/mmhg		Diastolic blood pressure/mmhg		Heart beat per/min.		Breath holding cap. (sec.)	
	PRE	POST	PRE	POST	PRE	POST	PRE	POST
1	119	117	81	76	72	68	50.77	59.45
2	121	119	78	78	68	62	47.73	54.72
3	117	118	78	74	64	62	51.46	56.95
4	112	116	75	76	70	68	43.28	47.58
5	120	118	80	79	72	64	38.96	44.76
6	116	119	78	80	62	60	62.13	64.27
7	113	114	75	76	66	62	44.91	48.65
8	122	118	76	78	70	64	52.14	56.76
9	118	116	77	74	66	62	49.12	56.23
10	124	118	81	76	76	72	35.91	38.46
11	119	116	73	72	64	62	33.65	45.12
12	121	120	77	75	62	58	39.07	41.64
13	114	118	72	74	74	70	49.73	52.15
14	118	114	80	79	66	60	37.92	39.64
15	121	116	82	79	74	70	52.15	62.15
16	117	116	72	74	62	60	47.18	56.94
17	119	118	78	76	64	60	60.7	66.42
18	123	120	76	74	74	70	49.05	54.68
19	120	118	75	76	72	68	33.79	36.81
20	123	119	79	75	60	62	39.22	42.61
21	116	116	75	76	70	64	42.71	51.08
22	123	120	78	75	66	64	53.69	59.46
23	**114**	**118**	**74**	**78**	**64**	66	33.77	39.19
24	**121**	**119**	**76**	**72**	**68**	62	38.87	34.65
25	**116**	**117**	**82**	**79**	**70**	62	63.53	70.52

GROUP-C

(ASANA &PRANAYAMA MIX GROUP)

PHYSIOLOGICAL VARIABLES

Subjects	Systolic blood pressure/mmhg		Diastolic blood pressure/mmhg		Heart beat per/min.		Breath holding cap. (sec.)	
	PRE	POST	PRE	POST	PRE	POST	PRE	POST
1	119	117	75	78	66	62	43.89	49.58
2	120	118	78	74	68	64	37.48	41.25
3	117	119	80	77	74	68	46.11	47.56
4	121	118	76	80	66	66	49.36	52.68
5	122	116	76	78	78	70	36.19	37.15
6	117	118	74	73	64	66	42.66	44.56
7	120	117	81	76	68	64	58.18	62.15
8	123	120	78	76	70	62	32.77	36.84
9	117	119	72	76	62	62	34.67	39.54
10	119	117	77	80	62	58	39.5	45.65
11	116	117	75	76	68	64	44.13	50.79
12	118	120	79	80	64	66	48.11	54.46
13	120	118	80	76	76	72	47.18	58.34
14	124	118	83	76	70	66	40.12	45.62
15	118	114	76	74	74	64	38.69	46.32
16	116	119	78	78	68	66	42.19	42.09
17	115	118	71	75	62	58	48.56	47.65
18	118	114	78	72	68	64	59.71	64.29
19	122	121	76	74	78	72	42.48	48.28
20	116	118	78	76	64	62	49.18	49.25
21	125	120	82	74	78	74	44.17	53.25
22	119	117	83	80	76	72	49.15	49.76
23	114	116	78	79	72	70	43.83	44.38
24	118	114	81	74	76	70	38.28	47.65
25	120	116	77	72	68	68	31.37	38.54

GROUP-D

(CONTROL GROUP)

PHYSIOLOGICAL VARIABLES

Subjects	Systolic blood pressure/mmhg		Diastolic blood pressure/mmhg		Heart beat per/min.		Breath holding cap. (sec.)	
	PRE	POST	PRE	POST	PRE	POST	PRE	POST
1	118	116	76	75	72	72	51.48	52.06
2	122	123	80	82	66	68	42.12	38.97
3	117	119	74	73	70	66	38.49	39.56
4	123	120	78	76	78	74	44.13	46.18
5	114	117	75	77	66	68	35.36	37.68
6	120	119	82	79	74	72	38.18	33.54
7	116	116	71	72	62	64	50.63	51.21
8	115	118	73	75	68	70	43.16	39.84
9	118	120	78	76	70	74	36.73	40.69
10	123	119	81	78	64	66	46.21	45.27
11	120	118	74	76	68	64	53.15	52.96
12	122	120	78	78	62	66	35.12	35.79
13	116	118	72	74	76	74	39.73	38.24
14	117	115	79	75	78	70	44.18	40.85
15	123	121	76	80	64	66	51.69	53.74
16	121	122	75	78	68	70	34.83	37.95
17	117	114	79	74	70	74	59.87	56.08
18	119	118	73	74	72	74	32.65	35.83
19	117	119	78	79	60	66	52.28	51.76
20	118	121	80	80	62	64	46.16	42.8
21	124	121	76	74	76	72	34.87	36.49
22	118	119	78	76	58	62	36.53	42.91
23	114	116	72	76	62	64	47.49	44.36
24	116	114	79	75	68	64	65.48	68.46
25	118	119	75	78	64	66	49.53	47.64

GROUP-A

(YOG ASANA)

HAEMATOLOGICAL

Subjects	WBC (10^3/ul)		RBC (10^6/ul)		HEMOGLOBIN (g/dl)		PLATLETS (10^3/ul)	
	PRE	POST	PRE	POST	PRE	POST	PRE	POST
1	7.6	11.1	5.51	5.19	13.2	13	214	253
2	6.7	6.9	4.9	4.42	13.9	13.2	252	247
3	5.1	5	4.58	4.3	11.9	11.5	318	279
4	7.6	6.4	3.16	5.34	9.1	12.4	289	246
5	4.6	5.7	5.16	5.08	13	12.9	303	330
6	8.2	9.3	5	3.92	12.9	10.5	269	281
7	6.5	5.3	4.45	4.79	11.4	11.8	315	266
8	5.5	6.6	4.55	4.66	12	11.9	293	286
9	6.5	7.6	3.65	3.64	10.9	11.1	252	221
10	8	7.3	4.43	3.83	9.1	11.9	456	375
11	6.4	5.8	4.46	4.76	10.4	10.7	285	301
12	6.1	7.6	3.62	5.01	9.4	13.2	268	293
13	7.5	7	3.67	3.39	10.6	10.4	268	216
14	5.1	5.3	4.46	4.32	10.6	11	308	353
15	6.3	6.3	4.15	4.58	10.1	13	325	267
16	7.8	6.5	4.48	4.5	12	13	207	285
17	7.7	7	4.4	4.38	11.5	11.6	262	285
18	6.8	7.8	3.48	5.36	9.8	13.8	345	278
19	7	7.4	4.91	5.17	12.8	13.2	354	342
20	5.5	4.2	4.55	4.46	11.2	11.7	281	229
21	8.3	6.4	5.15	5.15	11.2	11.7	236	248
22	6.2	6.2	4.21	4.31	10.3	10.8	318	274
23	10.4	8.7	4.88	4.85	7.8	11.9	261	301
24	7.7	7.3	4.08	4.08	12.6	13.5	340	303
25	7.6	7.3	4.58	4.53	13	13.4	273	261

GROUP-B

(PRANAYAMA)

HAEMATOLOGICAL

Sr No	WBC (10^3/ul)		RBC (10^6/ul)		HEMOGLOBIN (g/dl)		PLATLETS (10^3/ul)	
	PRE	POST	PRE	POST	PRE	POST	PRE	POST
1	6.4	6.3	4.56	4.7	11	12	252	253
2	6.8	8.8	4.56	4.08	12	11.7	237	248
3	6.4	7.6	3.92	3.74	12	12.1	212	275
4	8.5	7.3	5.42	5.12	13.4	13.8	210	230
5	10.6	8.1	5.27	5.23	12.6	12.9	283	293
6	6.1	5.9	5.52	5.51	13.3	13.9	397	302
7	6.5	6.2	4.5	3.82	11.6	10.9	323	279
8	6.9	11.2	4.82	5.08	10.2	14.5	329	386
9	5.3	6.3	4.61	4.69	11.9	12	298	341
10	6.7	8.2	4.86	5.05	12.6	13.4	454	419
11	6.9	5.8	3.49	3.68	10.2	11	314	249
12	9.5	7.5	3.96	3.71	10.2	9.7	239	285
13	5.3	12.9	3.83	5.16	9.9	12.9	263	428
14	6.8	5.5	4.06	3.29	11.7	10.6	194	218
15	5.9	5.4	4.03	4.44	6.3	11.8	228	272
16	5.1	6.9	3.75	3.85	10.3	11.2	277	237
17	9.8	10.2	4.61	3.92	11.2	9.9	217	267
18	8.8	8.3	4.14	4.52	11.2	12.6	342	312
19	7	8.4	4.01	4.71	10.2	12	377	232
20	7.6	7.1	5.04	5.26	10.8	11.6	293	230
21	7.8	4.8	4.89	4.43	11.9	12.2	348	264
22	7	8.8	4.57	4.79	11.4	12	353	276
23	7.5	**4.8**	7.01	**4.59**	11.9	12.7	328	215
24	8.8	**4.2**	4.72	**5.23**	11.5	11.4	272	204
25	11.3	**9.7**	4.34	**4.99**	11	12.7	214	198

GROUP-C

ASANA & PRANAYAMA)

HAEMATOLOGICAL

Subjects	WBC (10^3/ul)		RBC (10^6/ul)		HEMOGLOBIN (g/dl)		PLATLETS (10^3/ul)	
	PRE	POST	PRE	POST	PRE	POST	PRE	POST
1	8.2	7.8	4.93	5.02	12.09	13.4	196	225
2	10	11.4	4.87	4.9	13.9	13.7	223	229
3	5.2	4.1	4.57	4.69	11.5	11.9	228	220
4	7	7.5	4.25	4.41	11	11.6	268	310
5	8.4	8.1	4.42	4.99	12.5	14	408	412
6	5.3	9.6	4.31	4.86	10.4	10.6	264	311
7	6.2	9.3	4.65	4.71	11.9	11.9	240	258
8	5.3	6.8	3.8	4.22	9.2	10.3	186	313
9	8.3	6.7	4.57	4.29	11.5	11.3	225	282
10	6.8	7.5	4.48	4.58	10.6	12.7	260	247
11	5.2	4.9	4.3	4.49	10.9	10.9	269	202
12	6	7.5	3.74	4.26	10.4	12.4	340	328
13	5.7	7.3	4.55	4.2	10.4	11.5	303	248
14	7.2	5.5	3.92	4.38	11.3	12	292	278
15	8.6	8.4	4.95	5.12	11.8	12.7	319	336
16	8.2	5.6	4.83	4.79	10.5	10.6	246	260
17	6	7.1	4.35	4.49	11.2	13.6	235	255
18	7.8	6	4.21	3.9	11.2	11.9	249	275
19	5.3	5.5	4.59	4.86	12	13.1	381	236
20	6.6	6.9	5.32	4.54	8.8	11.1	409	335
21	7.5	9	5.09	5.51	11.9	12.6	309	293
22	10.3	7.9	4.53	4.76	12	13.2	257	288
23	8.7	8.6	4.7	4.68	12.4	13.6	252	277
24	6	8	4	4.87	11.4	13.9	265	240
25	7.1	8.2	4.34	4.44	11.1	12	307	292

GROUP-D

CONTROL GROUP

HAEMATOLOGICAL

subjects	WBC (10^3/ul)		RBC (10^6/ul)		HEMOGLOBIN (g/dl)		PLATLETS (10^3/ul)	
	PRE	POST	PRE	POST	PRE	POST	PRE	POST
1	5.1	3.8	4.46	4.16	12.9	12.7	204	178
2	8.8	8.3	4.83	4.99	12.5	13.6	335	308
3	6.2	9.2	4.53	4.34	12	12.1	287	222
4	10.4	12.7	5.05	5.42	13.8	15.4	331	357
5	6.9	6.3	4.67	4.26	12.5	11.9	400	391
6	7.5	8.7	4.15	4.76	9.8	12.2	384	253
7	8.8	12.3	5	4.9	13.4	12.4	218	255
8	5.5	5.1	3.47	3.81	10.2	11.3	250	355
9	7	5.7	4.37	4.69	10.6	11.8	255	200
10	8.3	7.2	4.75	4.69	12.8	12.2	363	390
11	7.9	7.7	4.66	4.66	11	10.6	269	236
12	8.5	9.8	4.84	4.32	12.6	11.6	352	401
13	8.1	6.7	4.85	4.58	11.8	11.7	541	394
14	8.7	8.8	4.72	4.32	12.7	12.9	473	409
15	6.3	7.7	4.68	4.23	12	11.2	289	152
16	11	8.8	4.65	4.39	12.3	11.6	408	373
17	5.4	5.3	4.27	4.1	11.3	11.2	190	242
18	8.4	6.6	4.46	4.68	11.7	12.6	169	193
19	6.4	4.7	4.49	5.19	9.2	11	406	268
20	6.5	8.1	4.91	5.34	10.5	13.2	237	231
21	8.2	6.9	4.3	4.78	10.1	11.3	253	272
22	7.2	9.1	4.89	4.13	12.3	13.1	274	270
23	5	5.5	3.91	4.32	9.7	11.2	385	318
24	8.4	4.7	3.69	3.71	10.1	10.4	249	221
25	6.4	5.5	5.01	5.17	13.6	14.36	212	241

RESEARCH REVIEW JOURNALS Volume-04 Issue-06 June-2019

ISSN: 2455-3085 (Online)
RESEARCH REVIEW International Journal of Multidisciplinary
www.rrjournals.com[UGC Listed Journal]

Effect of Yoga Asana Training on Physical Fitness Variables of School Level Students

[1]Shiv Kant & [2]Dr. Amarjit Kaur

[1]Research scholar, Department of Physical Education, Panjab University, Chandigarh (India)
[2]Professor in Physical Education, Govind National College, Narangwal, (Ludhiana) (India)

ARTICLE DETAILS

Article History
Published Online: 12 June 2019

Keywords
Yoga Asana, Physical fitness, Strength, Flexibility, Agility, Speed, Endurance..

ABSTRACT

The purpose of the study was found out the effects of yoga asanas training on physical fitness of school level students. This is an experimental study. For achieving the purpose of the study 50 male students of 9th to 12th classes from Govt. senior secondary school were selected as the subjects of the study. They were divided into two groups randomly, each group have 25 subjects. Group-I given Yoga Asana training, Group- II treated as a control group. Control group was not participated any type of yoga program. Strength, agility, speed, flexibility and endurance were selected as the variables of physical fitness for the study. The subjects were participated in six weeks Yoga Asanas training program. The data for the study was collected through the pre and post-test of six weeks training program. For analyzing the data of physical fitness variables descriptive analysis and t- test was applied at 0.05 level of significant. The result of the study showed that there was a significant effect of Yoga Asana training on physical fitness variables.

1. Introduction

In present time Physical fitness level of students become a big problem. In modern scientific life we easily access of everything and hardly do physical labor. This is a "push-button" age. In this modern world man has become idle and sedentary. We are not aware about physical activities and health program. This physical inactivity creates many health problems for us. It's not affected only our health but also our social life. Physical inactivity and negative social stigma are decreasing student's physical fitness. Students need of a good physical and mental fitness awareness to face the every problem of life. With physical and mental fitness they face challenges and making an achievement in any field of life.

Physical activity is the best tool to improve our health related quality of life. Physical fitness is must for every individual to function effectively in day to day life. We must exercise and physical active daily if want to be fit.

Yogic routine helps to attained fitness excellently. Yogic exercise deals with our inner and outer organs on which health depends upon. Different postures of yoga giving different movements to vital organs of our body. A continuous training of yoga is very beneficially for every aspect of life. It is very helpful for the proper fitness of body and mind. It's improving our flexibility and stamina for running. Yoga helps to maintaining cardiovascular system. it is very helpful to control disease, spiritual development and overcome from tension.

In this study we find out the effect of yoga on physical fitness variables of school level students.

2. Objectives of study:-

To find out the effect of yoga asana training on physical fitness variables.

3. Research Methodology:-

Selection of the subject

For the present study 50 male students of 9th to 12th classes from Govt. Senior Secondary School, Ugalan (Hisar), Haryana were selected by purposive sampling as the subjects of the study and they were divided into two groups randomly. Each group has 25 subjects. Group-I for Yoga Asana training group and Group- II treated as a Control Group. Physical fitness test were conducted of the both groups before the of Yoga Asana training program. Group-I given six weeks, five days a week training program of Yoga Asana whereas Control group was not participated any type of specific training program, those given only general exercises. At the end of six weeks training program physical fitness test components were conducted on both groups.

Selection of test

The purpose of this study was to test the effect of Yoga Asana on physical fitness, the following test items was selected to measure the physical fitness components.

1. Speed – 50 meter dash running
2. Strength – Standing broad jump
3. Endurance - 12 Minutes walk /run
4. Flexibility – Sit and Reach
5. Agility – Shuttle run

Experimental design and training Schedule

This is an experiment design study. In this study pre test were conducted prior to Yoga Asana training program of six weeks, five day in a week and post tests were conducted after the training program. Each training session was 50 minutes duration. Each session had 10 minutes warming up and 10 minutes cooling down exercises. Total 10 Asanas were includes in this training program. Each asana was repeated by three times. The name of Asana is as follows

- *Tadasana*
- *Trikonasana*
- *Padmasana*
- *Vajrasana*
- *Bhujangasana*
- *Shalabasana*
- *Dhanurasana*
- *Halasana*
- *Chakrasana*
- *Matsayasana*

Statistical procedure

For analyzed the effects of Yoga Asana training on Physical Fitness components a descriptive study analysis and t- test were used at level of significance 0.05. The result was showed in table.

4. Results of the Study:-

Table 2

Comparison of physical fitness level of Pre and Post results of experimental group and control group.

	Variable	Mean	Std. Deviation	Std. Error Mean	Std. Error Mean	T
Pre Experiment	50 Mts Dash (N=25)	8.1292	.72414	.14483	.20129	.238
		8.1772	.74263	.14853		
Post Experiment	50 Mts Dash (N=25)	7.6880	.73787	.14757	.20974	2.245
		8.1588	.75829	.15166		
Pre Experiment	Standing Broad Jump (N=25)	1.7176	.20809	.04162	.06151	1.262
		1.7952	.22420	.04484		
Post Experiment	Standing Broad Jump (N=25)	1.8580	.19719	.03944	.05571	.962
		1.8044	.22875	.04575		
Pre Experiment	Shuttle Run (N=25)	11.6508	.50512	.11302	.18113	1.976
		12.0088	.68820	.13764		
Post Experiment	Shuttle Run (N=25)	11.0360	.61417	.12283	.18728	4.912
		11.9560	.69973	.13995		
Pre Experiment	Sit and Reach (N=25)	7.2800	4.43959	.88792	1.27541	1.255
		5.6800	4.44147	.88829		
Post Experiment	Sit and Reach (N=25)	9.4800	4.21426	.84285	1.35366	2.719
		5.8000	4.65475	.93095		
Pre Experiment	12 minutes run/walk (N=25)	1852.0000	236.36131	47.27226	49.66447	1.240
		1790.4000	167.14465	33.42893		
Post Experiment	12 minutes run/walk	1913.6000	253.09550	50.61910	50.91012	2.499
		1786.4000	157.02654	31.40531		

The table showed the mean and SD and t value of physical fitness level of Experimental group and control group. The results of the data showed that pre experiment t value of 50 meters, Standing Broad jump Sit and reach and 12 minutes run/walk not significant, whereas t value of post experiment of 50 meters, Standing Broad jump Sit and reach and 12 minutes run/walk significant, the results of shuttle run is showed significant difference, but t value of post test almost double Which showed the there is significant improvement in physical fitness after 6 weeks Yoga Asana training and Yoga Asana recommended exercise for improvement of Physical fitness of school going students.

5. Conclusion

The results of the study clearly showed that the effects of yoga asanas training on school level students were positively significant. The results proved that yoga asanas are very helpful to improve physical fitness of the students.

References

1. Acharya BK., (2010), "Effect of Pranayama(voluntary regulated breathing) and Yogasana (yoga postures) on Lipid Profile in Normal Healthy Junior Footballers. *International Journal of Yoga.*
2. Anand BK. Yoga and medical sciences, (1976). Seminar on Yoga, science and man. *Central council for research in Indian Medicine and Homeopathy. New Delhi.*
3. Bhargava, R. Gogate, M.G. and Mascarenhas, J.F. (1988) "Autonomic responses to breath holding and its variations following pranayama". *Dissertation abstract international.*
4. Chen TL, Mao HC, Lai CH, Li CY, Kuo CH.(2009) The effect of yoga exercise intervention on health related physical fitness. *In school-age asthmatic children.*
5. Culos-Reed SN, Carlson LE, Daroux LM, Hately-Aldous S.(2005). A pilot study of yoga for breast cancer survivors: physical and physiological benefits. *Psycho-Oncology. Epublished ahead of print on December.*
6. Dutta, Uma. (1990). " Effectiveness of General and Specific Streching Exerices on Flexibility in Gymnastics". *Abstract Cum Souvenir VI national conference and Seminar on Physical Education and Sports Science.*
7. Fondran Kristine M. (2008). The effect of Surya Namaskara yog practice on resting heart rate and blood pressure, flexibility, upper body muscle endurance and perceived well-being in healthy adults . *Cleveland state university.*
8. Ganguly, S.K. and Gharote, M.L.(1984). "Cardiovascular efficiency before and after yogic training". *Yoga mimamsa.*
9. Gedder M, Dolers.(1968.) "Effect of mobility patterning technique upon selected motor skill of primay school educate mentally retarded children". *The Research Quarterly 3913:953.*
10. Gharote, M.L., Ganguly, S.K. and Moorthy, A.M.(1976) "Effect of Yogic Training of Minimum Fitness". *Yoga Mimamsa 3&4:1-20.*

RESEARCH REVIEW JOURNALS

RESEARCH REVIEW
International Journal of Multidisciplinary

e-ISSN: 2455-3085
Impact Factor: 5.164 [SJIF]

ज्ञान-विज्ञान विमुक्तये

UGC Approved Journal
Journal No.: 44945

Journal is Indexed in
Google Scholar, IIJIF, SJIFactor, RESEARCH BIBLE, DRJI, GIF, UGC, Zenodo, Researcher ID [by Thomson Reutors]

Issued w.e.f. Nov-2018 Issue

CERTIFICATE OF PUBLICATION

This is to certify that Research Paper/ Article/ Case Paper entitled

Effect of Yoga Asana Training on Physical Fitness Variables of School Level Students

Authored By

Shiv Kant & Dr. Amarjit Kaur

has been published in Volume-4 | Issue-06 | June-2019 in this International Peer Reviewed ISSN Indexed Online Research Journal.

Ref. No. RRJ20190406318
Issued Date: 12-Jun-2019
editor.rrjournals@gmail.com
www.rrjournals.com
Certificate Verification visit: http://rrjournals.com/View-Certificate

RESEARCH REVIEW JOURNALS eISSN 2455-3085 AHMEDABAD

Chief Editor

ज्ञान-विज्ञान विमुक्तये

UGC Sponsored

3rd National Conference on Latest Trends in Health & Physical Education

Organized by:

University college of Medical Science

20th - 21st , August 2019

In Association with:

DASC SOCIETY

CERTIFICATE

This is to certify that,

Prof./Dr./Mrs./Mr./Ms. Shiv Kant

from Dept. of Physical Education. Panjab University. Chandigarh

Participated in the 3rd National Conference on Latest Trends in Health & Physical Education on 20th- 21st August 2019 as Delegates / Chairperson at UNIVERSITY COLLEGE OF MEDICAL SCIENCES (UNIVERSITY OF DELHI) He /She presented the paper (s) entitled EFFECT OF PRANAYAMA TRAINING ON PHYSIOLOGICAL VARIABLES OF SCHOOL LEVEL STUDENTS

DASC

SOCIETY

Strengthening Nation Through Sports

Prof. B.D. Banerjee
Patron & Staff Advisor
(Physical Education)

Dr. R. Chakravarty
Org. Secretary
LTHPE, 2019

MANIPAL UNIVERSITY JAIPUR

Department of Science and Technology

International Conference on Physical Education and Sports Science (ICPESS 20)

(Sponsored by Department of Science & Technology, Govt. of Rajasthan)

January 9-11, 2020

Organized by

Department of Arts (Physical Education)
Manipal University Jaipur

This is to certify that Ms./Mr./Dr. Shiv Kant

from Punjab University, Chandigarh presented a paper / made a poster presentation

titled Effect of hatha yoga on physical fitness variables on school students.

in the ICPESS 20, held at Manipal University Jaipur.

Prof Mridul Srivastava

Dr. Rina Poonia

Sr. No. 015

क्रीडा-भारती

NATIONAL SEMINAR

on

"Weight Management through Exercise & Yoga"

12th January, 2020

Organized by
Department of Physical Education
Chaudhary Bansi Lal University,
Bhiwani, Haryana

In Collaboration with
Kreeda Bharati, Bhiwani
Haryana

CERTIFICATE

This is to certify that

Dr./Mr./Mrs./ Shivkant (Res. Schoolar) From Punjab Univ. Chandigarh

has participated in the National Seminar "Weight Management through Exercise & Yoga" as a delegated and chaired a session/delivered a talk as a keynote speaker/presented a paper entitled Effect of Yoga Asana and Pranayama mix training on physical fitness variables of school level students held at the department of Physical Education, Chaudhary Bansi Lal University, Bhiwani **12th January, 2020**.

Dr. Suresh Kumar Malik
Convener

Dr. Anurag Sachan
Organizing Secretary

National Seminar on Sports Training

Organized by

Directorate of Sports, Panjab University, Chandigarh

January 12, 2017

CERTIFICATE

This is to certify that ZHN KANT

has participated/delivered lecture/chaired session/presented paper entitled YOGA FOR SPORTS PERFORMANCE in National Seminar on Sports Training held on January 12, 2017 organized by Directorate of Sports, Panjab University, Chandigarh.

Dr. Parminder Singh Ahluwalia
Patron

Dr. Rakesh Malik
Organizing Secretary

CHAPTER–V

SUMMARY, FINDINGS, CONCLUSIONS AND RECOMMENDATIONS

SUMMARY

Yoga is mixture of spiritual, mental and physical practice or tradition which originates in ancient India. Yogic practice has an excellent effect on physical and physiological parameters as per the previous research shown. A lot of space for the research is available in the field of Yoga with different parameters.

In the Present study four groups were randomly formed. Each group consists of 25 participants. The first group take part in Yoga Asana training, second groups was taking Pranayama training, third groups was performing mixture of yoga asana and pranayama training while the fourth groups act as control groups who did not take part in any training. Pretest and posttest was taken before and after the training provided of all groups including control group. To find out the best training method in comparison of control group analysis of co-variance was used as a part of general liner modal. The pretest was act as covariate for the present study. Physical, Physiological and Hematological variables were selected as dependent variables of the study while, the different training schedules were considered as independent variable for the present study.

The findings of the current study shows that various yoga trainings were significantly effective on physical fitness components like speed, strength, flexibility, endurance and agility and positively significant on physiological parameters like resting heart rate and breath holding capacity but not significant effect on blood pressure and except hemoglobin all hematological variables of the subjects.

FINDINGS

Following findings were observed after analysis the meaningful outcomes on the basis of attained data after the training provided.

FINDINGS IN PHYSICAL COMPONENTS

1. The pre-test and post-test mean comparison of speed produced highly significant results for Group A (Yoga Asana), Group B (Pranayama) and Group C (Yoga Asana and Pranayama mixed) training groups. But pre and post intervention mean comparison of Group D was non-significant (p-0.100) for speed. It was seen that all three trainings significantly improved the speed of students.
2. It was observed that the calculated value of F for group's interaction was 17.309 which were statistically significant at 0.05 level of alpha. The adjusted mean significantly varied among the groups after covariate the pretest. Maximum mean difference (0.502) was observed for Group C while paired sample t-test. and even the adjusted mean for post-test was minimum (M-7.71 seconds) for Group C compared to other groups indicating Yoga Asana and Pranayama mixed training best for speed.
3. Strength among students increased after three yoga trainings highly significantly. But non-significant improvement was noticed in control group.
4. The F value 31.775 for group's interaction illustrates significant difference in post intervention of Standing Broad Jump between the selected groups significant variation among the groups after covariate the pretest. With maximum adjusted mean (1.92m) Yoga asana proved best training for strength.
5. While assessing agility the mean time for training groups was significantly lower than pre-test contrarily in control group it non-significantly increased during post-test.
6. The adjusted mean were significantly different among the groups after covariate the pretest. In Group C maximum mean decrease was observed also adjusted mean was lowest with Yoga asana and pranayama mixed training proving it best for agility.
7. Flexibility of students increased during post-test but except control group(p-0.195) for all groups highly significant(p-0,000) p-value was calculated.
8. For Flexibility calculated value of F for group's interaction was 41.298 which were statistically significant. Yoga asana was found most impactful among all for flexibility with maximum adjusted mean 9.57.

9. It was observed during post-test that endurance among all training groups enhanced significantly but decline was seen in Control group.
10. The F value illustrates significant difference in endurance during post intervention of 12 Minute Run and Walk between the selected groups. Adjusted mean for mixed training was maximum (M-1968.7) showing it best among all for endurance.

FINDINGS IN PHYSIOLOGICAL VARIABLES

1. After 12 week training all study groups were showing decreased Systolic Blood pressure. It was seen that SBP decreased significantly with training in Group B (pranayama) and Group C(mixed).
2. It was observed that the calculated value of F for group's interaction was 1.871 which was not statistically significant at 0.05 level of alpha. Yoga asana and pranayama mixed training succeeded in controlling SBP more significantly with mean difference 1.400 and adjusted mean 117.39.
3. The effect of training on Diastolic Blood Pressure was visible in all the groups but significant impact was seen in Group B(Pranayama). The mean difference before and after intervention was maximum(1.520) for Group C(Yoga asana and pranayama).
4. It was observed that adjusted mean did not significantly varied among the groups after covariate the pretest. Rather maximum effect was seen with least adjusted mean (M-75.96) in Group C(Yoga asana and pranayama).
5. Significant decline in Heart rate of training groups was noticed during post-test but it increased for Group D(Control group). Group B(Pranayama) more efficiently improved heart rate of students with mean difference 3.760.
6. The adjusted mean significantly varied among the groups after covariate the pretest. Group B(Pranayama) having minimum adjusted mean(M-64.53) was more suitable training for heart rate.
7. Breath holding capacity of students improved with all training significantly but non-significantly in control group. Group B(Pranayama) had improved the breath holding of capacity of students most with 5.178 mean difference.

8. Significant difference in post intervention of Breath Holding Capacity between the selected groups after adjusted the covariate pretest of respective variable was observed. Highest adjusted mean (M-51.06) in Group B displayed the crucial role of Pranayama for improving breath holding capacity.

FINDINGS IN HEMATOLOGICAL VARIABLE

1. From the observations non-significant changes in White Blood Cells were noticed for all three training groups as well as control group. Where students in Group B and Group C had increased mean WBC, Group A had slight decline but Group D (Control) had larger decline in WBC.
2. It was observed that the calculated value of F for group's interaction was 0.287 indicating not significant variation among the groups. Largest increase in Group C (M-7.48) indicates that Yoga asana and pranayama mixed training is perfect for increasing WBC.
3. Except Group B, with non-significant but decreased, all other groups had non-significantly increased level of Red Blood Cells in post-test. Larger increase was noticed in mixed training group.
4. The F value 0.395 illustrates not significant difference in post intervention of Red Blood Cells between the selected groups after adjusted the covariate pretest of respective variable. With highest adjusted mean (M-4.64) yoga asana and pranayama mixed was found appropriate training for increased RBC.
5. Mean comparison between pre and post-test revealed significant difference in all groups for Hemoglobin. The great impact on hemoglobin was seen with yoga asana and pranayama mixed training having 0.984 highly significant mean difference.
6. Adjusted mean were not significantly varying among the groups after covariate the pretest. Group C (mixed training) was having highest adjusted mean(M-12.28) showing it more helpful for hemoglobin.
7. The results of the study revealed non-significant changes in Platelet count of students during pre-test and post-test. Maximum mean difference 13.640 was observed in Group B(Pranayama)

8. It was observed that the calculated value of F 0.186 illustrated non-significant difference in post intervention of Platelets between the selected groups after adjusted the covariate pretest of respective variable. Adjusted mean (M-285.62) was maximum resulted from yoga asana and pranayama mixed training.

The following findings given above were based on the outcomes of tables of between subjects factor which show the significant variation between different groups involved in the study. The brief description was given in the conclusions of the study the next main heading of this chapter.

CONCLUSIONS OF THE STUDY

The conclusion is proposed to help the reader comprehend why your research should matter to them afterward they have completed reading the thesis. A conclusion is not just a summary of your points or a re-statement of your research problem but a synthesis of key points.

1. It was concluded on the basis of the obtained outcomes that significance influence of Hath Yoga training on physical fitness variable was noticed after adjusted the mean values (covariate) therefore, the null hypothesis which was formulated earlier that "there is no significant difference in physical fitness variables on yoga asana group, pranayama group and asana pranayama combined group due to their respective hath yoga training with relatively control group" was not accepted. In Physical variables, Yoga asana was good for strength and flexibility but combined training of yoga asana and pranayama had effectively improved speed, agility and endurance among students.

2. In physiological variables the null hypothesis is falling to reject on some parameters for instance, diastolic and systolic blood pressure where training has similar effects. Whereas, resting heart rate and breath holding capacity has significant variation noticed after the given training. The Systolic blood pressure and Diastolic Blood Pressure showed positive impact of Yoga asana and pranayama mixed training but Pranayama was found most effective for heart rate and breath holding capacity.

3. In hematological variables all training groups have observed equal variance therefore, here; the researcher was failing to rejects the null hypothesis in each variable. Only hemoglobin increased significantly among all training groups after 12 weeks. Yoga asana and pranayama mixed training was found effective on all hematological variables like White Blood Cells, Red Blood Cells, Hemoglobin and platelets. Hematological parameters could be effected by various factors such as diet, rest, environment etc. which cannot be controlled properly during the training period. So, it may effects the results of the study that's why these factors should be considered as limitations of the study or beyond the control of the researcher.

RECOMMENDATIONS

Every research work has established some aim and objectives as per the nature of the study. The obtained consequences should bring meaningful and valuable phenomenon for the concerned population and society. These conclusions are important for our policy maker, social thinkers, govt. machineries who are responsible for betterment of sports environment in the nation. In the present study the following educational implications were suggested by the researcher on the basis of obtained consequences:

1. The yogic training should be implemented on the root level of the society for instance, in middle school to college or university level. Because these institutes are deals with the youth and healthy youth is the spine of every nation.
2. Yoga and physical education should be included in the curriculum of the each institute whether it should belong to engineering, science, medical science and art also.
3. The govt. authority should implement the means of yoga in each discipline of work to make the people healthy and fit and psychological wellbeing.
4. It is recommended that physical education teachers, trainers and coaches should give due importance to yoga and make it a part of their professional commitment.
5. New studies can be carried out to know the various effects of different yogic exercises combination.

6. Yoga, a form of mind- body work out, has become an increasingly well-known therapy used to maintain wellness, and alleviate a series of health problems and ailments. Yoga should be considered as a complementary treatment or alternative method for medical therapy in the treatment of different diseases.
7. Yoga suspends the fluctuations of the mind and by acting consciously, we live better and suffer less
8. Similar researcher can be conducted with different variables.
9. The experimental study should be more controlled in nature and scientific approach should as assessed.
10. The study should be conducted on different hematological parameters with different training plans.
11. Biomechanical analysis of Yogic movement can also be done
12. The present study was limited to male students only thus gender difference can be concluded only if females' students would be added.

CPSIA information can be obtained
at www.ICGtesting.com
Printed in the USA
LVHW012115291122
734192LV00014B/558

9 782177 100653